# DHEA:

## Unlocking the Secrets to the Fountain of Youth

### 2ND EDITION

## By Beth M. Ley with Richard N. Ash, M.D.

**BL Publications**
Aliso Viejo, CA

Ley, Beth M., 1964-
    DHEA: your responsibility: unlocking the secrets to the fountain of youth / by Beth M. Ley and Richard Ash.--2nd ed.
        p.  cm.
    Includes bibliographical references and index.
    ISBN 0-9642703-8-2
    1. Dehydroepiandrosterone--Physiological effect.
2. Dehydroepiandrosterone--Therapeutic use. 3. Aging--Endocrine aspects.    I. Ash, Richard, 1948-    . II. Title.
RM296.5.D45L49   1997
612.6'7--dc21                                                    97-22004
                                                                        CIP

Printed in the United States of America

First edition, January 1996.
Second edition, July 1997.

*DHEA: Your Responsibility, Unlocking the Secrets to The Fountain of Youth - 2nd edition* is not intended as medical advice. Its intention is solely informational and educational. It is wise to consult your doctor for any illness or medical condition.

**Credits:**
Various input provided: Samuel Yen, M.D., Stephen Langer, M.D., Bruce Hedendal, D.C., my parents, and especially my husband, Randy.

Artwork: Drawings-Stephanie Neesby Scott
Typesetting and Cover Design: BL Publications / Cuviello Creative Services, Palo Alto, CA.
Editing: Victoria Earhart, Ann Leaming, Sylvia Nelson

Additional languages available: German, Japanese, Spanish

# TABLE OF CONTENTS

*"In the next 30 years I fully expect to see life span of 120, 130 years in people who are completely intact. Technology now exists which can slow and perhaps even reverse significantly the physical deterioration and disease which are currently called aging."*

Dr. Ronald Klatz, M.D., President of the American
Academy of Anti-Aging Medicine

*"Recent studies have shown that supplementing with DHEA increases the lifespan of lab animals, prevents experimental cancers, improves immune functions... and probably helps prevent or reverse osteoporosis. Innovative clinicians are using DHEA successfully to treat inflammatory bowel disease, chronic fatigue syndrome, lupus erythematosus, and some manifestations of aging."*

*Townsend Letter For Doctors*

*"Ponce de Leon might still be here, in search of his fountain of youth, if he had run across DHEA."*

Dr. Julian Whitaker, M.D., *"Health and Healing"*

*"DHEA levels naturally drop as people age, and there is good reason to think that taking a DHEA supplement may extend your life and make you more youthful while you are alive. DHEA protects brain cells from Alzheimer's disease and other senility-associated degenerative conditions."*

Dr. Ward Dean, M.D., *"Smart Drugs and Nutrients"*

*"I strongly believe that using DHEA will improve your health and extend your life."*

Dr. Robert Atkins, M.D.

*"Current research suggests that DHEA may be of value in preventing and treating cardiovascular disease, high cholesterol, diabetes, obesity, cancer, Alzheimer's disease, other memory disturbances, immune system disorders including AIDS and chronic fatigue. DHEA may also enhance the body's immune response to viral and bacterial infections. Perhaps most interesting, DHEA is currently being investigated as an anti-aging hormone... New evidence suggest this hormone is so beneficial for so many different conditions that it may turn out to be the most important medical advance of the decade."*

Dr. Alan Gaby, M.D., *"Preventing and Reversing Osteoporosis"*

*DHEA increased the normal lifespan of lab animals by 50%, reduced body fat in overweight animals by one-third and increased lean muscle tissue."*

Dr. Arthur Schwartz, Temple University

*DHEA has an apparent ability to lower body weight regardless of caloric intake.*

Dr. Neecie Moore, *"Bountiful Health, Boundless Energy, Brilliant Youth, The Facts About DHEA"*

# AUTHOR PREFACE

When I began research for the first edition for this book, few people had even heard of DHEA as it was not available without a prescription. In October of 1994, the Health and Education Act changed the regulatory status of DHEA and by July of 1996, just about every supplement manufacture in the United States was introducing their own brand of DHEA and it is now readily available. We all have learned a great deal about DHEA in the last year, thus the need for revisions.

I realize much of this book is technical. I have tried to make the information understandable for the average reader. The purpose of this book is not to entertain, it is to educate. I am not willing to write in such simple language that you feel insulted. I feel that you and your intelligence deserve much more credit. If you are interested enough about your health and longevity to buy this book, you are obviously smart enough to read something written above third grade reading level.

I also want to comment on the use of laboratory animals used to conduct much of the research on DHEA. While I am against cruelty to animals of any kind (and have been a vegetarian for about 10 years), I realize that sometimes there is a need to use laboratory animals for the purposes of education.

Animals are a valuable experimental tool because they do not respond to the placebo effect which otherwise can greatly distort the research results. In humans, the average placebo response is over 60 percent, and may be as high as 100 percent. This, of course, is one of the reasons that a good valid human study should be a double-blind, cross-over study.

In addition, many, many years are required to fully examine the anti-aging effects of a substance in humans. The effects can be seen much faster in laboratory animals who have a normal lifespan of a few years compared to many decades in our case. I can only hope that the animals used in the experiments discussed in this book were not treated inhumanely.

Because so much has changed, and because we have learned so much in the last year since DHEA entered the market place, I felt a need to introduce a 2nd Edition the earlier version *DHEA: Unlocking The Secrets To The Fountain of Youth* to keep you up to date.

I invited Dr. Richard Ash, a prominent New York M.D., who has been using DHEA on his patients for several years, to work with me on this revision and share with us what he has learned about the use of DHEA and pregnenolone. His input has been invaluable, especially for two important chapters, "Taking DHEA Responsibly" and "DHEA Delivery Systems."

I decided to change the name of the book to reflect the new attitudes towards DHEA and other hormones. In spite of their safety, they must be used properly in order to avoid side effects. Used improperly, DHEA can be harmful just like all other substances, even water.

Just because DHEA and other "naturally occurring substances" including other hormones such as melatonin, pregnenolone, and androstenedione (sold as a precursor to testosterone), are now sold over the counter does not mean that they are totally safe. We are talking about **hormones; the chemicals which regulate all bodily functions**. They are not simple vitamins or minerals. They have powerful, drug-like effects on the body and require a degree of self- responsibility to use and obtain desirable, long term effects. This requires **self- education.** You cannot rely upon your doctor to give you good advice because over 95 percent of medical doctors know very little about DHEA and other such chemicals. When I told my doctor that I was taking DHEA, he told me that it was a placebo. Needless to say, I have switched doctors.

If you are dissatisfied with the care you are receiving from your current physician I strongly suggest you consider contacting the American College of Advancement in Medicine (ACAM) for a physician referral in your geographical area. You may call them toll free at 1-800-532-3688. This is a professional non-profit membership society dedicated to educating physicians on the latest findings and emerging procedures in preventative/nutritional medicine.

# INTRODUCTION

Our bodies are run by hormones. Most people know that hormones are responsible for our sexuality, give us our body shape, determine how much body hair we have, give our voice a high or low pitch, and our many other male and female attributes. But hormones also regulate our sleep, immune system, metabolic rate, body temperature, weight, appetite, mental state, moods, memory, and much more.

Hormones are also known to impact many human aging parameters. DHEA, short for dehydroepiandrosterone, produced by the adrenal glands, is the most abundant hormone in the body. It is a precursor to the sex hormones and a number of other hormones in the body. Levels of this amazing hormone are highest when we are in the prime of life, age 18-25, after which production gradually begins to slow down.

Current research suggests that DHEA may be of value in preventing and treating cardiovascular disease, high cholesterol, diabetes, osteoporosis, obesity, cancer, Alzheimer's disease, other memory deficits, immune system disorders including acquired immunodeficiency syndrome (AIDS), and chronic fatigue. DHEA may also enhance the body's immune response to viral and bacterial infections. Perhaps most interesting, DHEA is currently being investigated as an anti-aging hormone.

Studies show that an increase in blood levels of DHEA sulfate is associated with a 36 percent reduction in mortality from any cause. Studies also show that we can actually prevent disease if we can maintain high levels of DHEA! This book will explain how to do that... safely... without side effects. You will also find out about the potential of a special extract from wild yam.

Many of you have probably never even heard of DHEA - you probably were interested in the book because it promised to reveal the secret of youth and longevity. You will not be disappointed. Once you understand DHEA, you will understand the secret.

Yes, this does sound like DHEA is a miracle drug. DHEA may be a miracle, but it is not really a drug. It is a naturally occurring substance produced in our adrenal glands.

DHEA is widely used for a number of degenerative conditions. The use of DHEA has been highly effective in conditions such as AIDS, osteoporosis, to prevent cardiogenesis and to slow development of diabetes, atherosclerosis, hypertension, memory disorders, fat mobilization problems and cancer. Additional clinical trials are in progress in the areas of cancer, diabetes, obesity, hypercholesterolemia, Alzheimer's disease and multiple sclerosis.

While there are over 4,500 published papers on DHEA, most of these studies have been conducted on free form DHEA or the compound, DHEA-S. Few published clinical studies have been done on naturally derived compounds such as from Dioscorea which are promoted as DHEA precursors. This is not because these plant derived compounds do not have medicinal value, it is largely because such natural substances cannot be patented and pharmaceutical companies are more interested in patentable substances which lend them a greater ability to rapidly recoup their financial investment.

The purpose of this book is to inform you of this exciting pro-hormone, DHEA, and explain the significance of healthy DHEA levels in the body. This book will explain what lowers DHEA levels in the body and the possible implications of this decrease, and finally to tell you about the various benefits of supplemental DHEA and of natural phytochemicals so that you can determine if they can help you.

# STRESS, LIFE EXPECTANCY, DISEASE AND AGING

What is our true life expectancy and why do so many of us die so young?

Genesis 6:3 states, *"Then the Lord said, I will not allow people to live forever; they are mortal. From now on they will live no longer than 120 years."*

At the height of the Roman Empire, people only lived to be about 26 years old. At the turn of the century the average life expectancy for a U.S. male was 49 years. In 1991, the average life expectancy at birth in the U.S. reached 75.5 years. Today, it is no longer uncommon to see people doing very well at ages 80 and 90. Much of this is due to advances in medicine, surgery and drugs. We no longer have to worry about many of the diseases which previously ended life prematurely for many.

The oldest known person, Sharali Misimiv, was believed to be 168 years old. He lived in a remote Russian village in the state of Azerbaijan, where he died in 1973. The people of Abkhasia, the remote mountain region of southern Russia, were renowned for their longevity. Also from this area was the oldest known woman who reportedly died at age 140. In this area most people are simple field workers where there are few paved roads and other amenities of modern living. They credit their good health to exercise and light eating.

Another community famed for their longevity are the Hunzas who are said to live to be healthy, active and disease free, well past the age of 100. And there are other communities as well. All of these communities base their living on simplicity and wholesomeness. Their lives are uncomplicated and void of the stress that dominates so many of our lives. Most of us in the U.S. would think that these people are a couple hundred years behind the times and, also, very boring.

Some researchers suggest that the life expectancy of other animals can give us a rough idea of our own. The life expectancy of most other animals is roughly seven times the point at which they reach maturity. A medium size dog, for example, reaches full growth at around two years, the life expectancy is around 14. A horse reaches maturity about three, and lives to be 20 or 25. Rabbits can live to be seven years old, while they reach maturity at about 11 months. Hamsters live about five years and reach maturity at about eight months. In the wild, few animals die of "old age". The causes of death are many and varied.

Humans reach maturity around age 20. This, times seven equals 140 years. But most of us barely reach just half this age. Among humans it is much easier to determine cause of death. In 1992, the top causes of death were as follows:

1) Heart disease, 33%

2) Cancer, 23%

3) Strokes, 7%

4) Lung diseases, 4%

5) Accidents, 4%

6) Pneumonia / Flu, 4%

7) Diabetes, 2%

8) Suicide, 1.4%

9) AIDS, 1.4%

10) Homicide, 1.2%

11) Liver disease / Cirrhosis, 1.2%

12) Kidney disease, 1%

Almost every one of these can be largely prevented or at least postponed with proper diet and lifestyle habits. Alcohol use and abuse can contribute to heart disease, cancer, stroke, liver disease and even accidents. Smoking is a major contributor to many of these causes as well.

The quality of the time that we do live is every bit as important as the length. We can do more to ensure a better quality of life as we age. One out of three Americans will get cancer at some point in their life-time, and by the year 2000, that number is expected to rise to one out of two. Nearly 60% of all people over 65 years have high blood pressure, and nearly one-third have heart disease. Forty-five percent of the elderly are on prescription drugs for arthritis, hypertension, glaucoma, etc.

# Is Aging Normal?

We could probably safely answer "Yes," but we need to qualify it with, "to some extent". We know that aging and eventually death are inevitable, but why is it that so many people live longer and healthier lives than others? And how is it that some people seem "old" for their age, while others are "young" for their age?

We sometimes use the description, "she looks pretty good, for someone her age," but how do we know how someone should look at a certain age? Some people seem to do everything wrong; smoke, drink, eat a high-fat, low-fiber diet, don't exercise, yet live a long healthy life. Then there are those who seem to do everything right, and they die young of a heart attack. It doesn't make sense.

Aging is a natural biological process; however, predisposition to premature aging or death may be caused by an improper diet and bad habits. Aging may also, to some extent, depend on

13

genetics.

So what keeps us healthy? Our immune system. It protects us from anything harmful entering the body - bacteria, viruses, allergens, waste materials and even cancerous cells. As part of the immune system, the thymus, spleen, lymph nodes, white blood cells, bone marrow (where blood cells are made), antibodies, and interferon each have protective roles to keep us healthy.

Over time, abuse and overwork eventually take toll on these organs and glands and they begin to lose efficiency and effectiveness. As the immune system begins to break down one becomes more susceptible to infections and numerous health problems.

# Accelerated Aging

We know that aging is greatly accelerated with poor dietary habits and abuse to the body. How much of aging is predestined and how much is preventable and to what degree? The answers are largely dependent upon these two simplified categories: What we put into the body and what we don't put in it.

**1. What we put in:**
> "Junk" food - empty calories, sugar, saturated fat, etc.
> Alcohol, tobacco, nicotine, and other drugs
> Pollutants, carcinogens, free radical forming substances,
> > including ultraviolet rays from the sun.
> Stress (causing the adrenal glands to secrete adrenaline)

**2. What we don't put in**
> Adequate supplies of all vitamins, minerals, complex
> > carbohydrates, amino acids, fiber, water, trace
> > nutrients, enzymes, etc.
> Adequate supplies of antioxidants
> Adequate rest and relaxation
> Emotional well-being; peace and happiness
> Exercise

# Hormones and Aging

Hormones are known to impact many human aging parameters. Certainly everyone is familiar with menopause, but contemporary researchers are beginning to explore the male equivalent of menopause, called "andropause," as well as an endocrine transition that occur in both sexes, "adrenopause." Growth hormone secretion also declines with age, affecting muscle mass and vigor.

Many individuals are genetically programmed for a susceptibility to decline in thyroid function or insulin resistance. The hypothalamus, pituitary, testes and ovaries, adrenal, pancreas, and thyroid participate in a complexly orchestrated process. Intervention aimed at selectively retarding certain features of aging must strive to avoid creating system imbalance. Endocrine aging affects skin, hair, body-fat composition, muscles, bones, liver, brain function, sleep, digestion, the cardiovascular system, and numerous other systems and functions.

Outside the intricate network of feedback loops that comprises the primary endocrine system is a mysterious gland that may play the most important role of all in "pacing" the aging process: the pineal. Studies of melatonin administration in animals show that it has a profound life-extending effect.

Hormone replacement therapy implicated to retard aging include:

1. Estrogen and progesterone
2. Testosterone
3. Dehydroepiandrosterone (DHEA)
4. Thyroid hormone
5. Growth hormone
6. Melatonin
7. Pregnenolone (Precursor to DHEA)

# Hormonal Effects

Hormone production and release is regulated by other hormones; by nerve signals and by signals from the target organ. Information regarding each hormone level is fed back to the originating gland which then responds accordingly.

This self-regulation method, termed biofeedback, is extremely precise in maintaining balance among each and every circulating hormone. Excess amounts of any one hormone, or inadequate amounts of another, disrupt the balance creating symptoms such as:

| | |
|---|---|
| PMS | Acne |
| Sleep disturbances | Fatigue |
| Depression | Headaches |
| Unwanted hair growth | Weight gain |
| Water retention | Breast swelling |
| Fibrocystic breasts | Loss of libido |
| Heavy or irregular menses | Uterine fibroid |
| Cravings for sweets, and many more | |

Supplemental synthetic hormones are not subject to the normal metabolic control of the body. Thus, their effects can not be turned off or tuned down through the counter balance of other hormones. (These synthetic compounds also cannot be excreted by the normal means.)

Synthetic hormones are by no means equivalent to natural hormones produced in the body. Hormone balance is completely destroyed by the introduction of synthetics. This is the major difference between natural hormones and those synthetically produced and introduced to the body.

The cycle of rest and activity in lower animals is dictated by instinct which is largely moderated by hormones. Mating, eating, sleeping, hibernation, migration, etc., are moderated by hormones and hormonal changes in the body.

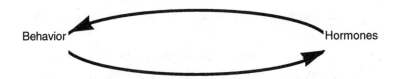

Behavior ← → Hormones

Animals react to feelings or instinct, but humans are free to override these feelings. If we choose to do so we then hasten aging. If we feel tired, instead of napping, we drink coffee or other caffeine containing beverages, or take energy-boosting supplements, or smoke cigarettes.

## Typical Behavior Response

| Stimuli | Animals | Humans |
|---------|---------|--------|
| **Fatigue** | Sleep | Drink coffee, cola or other caffeine-containing beverage |
| | | Smoke a cigarette |
| | | Eat, often sweets or high fat snack foods |
| **Boredom** | Play | Eat, drink, smoke, watch TV |
| **Hunger** | Hunt, and eat until satiated | Eat, until over-stuffed |

## Preserving the Balance

Beginning with our genetic material (DNA and RNA) and the enzymes they produce, our cells team with molecules that react with precise order. Each of the cells in the body are made up of molecules that found their proper place because DNA directed them there.

The body makes its messages known by producing molecules that can carry the messages. The message carriers are hormones.

Just the smell of food being prepared stimulates the digestive process in the body. You may not have even realized that you were hungry until you detected the aroma of food being prepared close by. Sometimes it's just the thought of eating that stimulates the digestive process.

The presence of food in our mouths automatically triggers the digestive processes. If you bite into a lemon, the juice instantly makes your mouth water as salivary glands under your tongue start secreting two digestive enzymes, salivary amylase and maltase. If you even think about biting into a lemon, your mouth waters and the same salivary enzymes are produced, even though there is nothing to digest. The message sent from the brain can be even more important than the presence of actual food. Words and images function just as well as "real" molecules to trigger the ongoing process of life.

Emotions can be transformed into molecules of adrenaline rushing through your bloodstream. These, in turn, activate receptors situated on the outside of your heart cells, which, in turn, tell each cell that it is appropriate to twitch faster than normal.

# Effects of Stress on Aging

We are all too familiar with stress. We are told to avoid it. We are told stress is not good for us. Stress is defined as any emotional, physical, social, ecological, economic, or other factor that requires a bodily response or change. Our society inflicts multitudinous stresses, both external and internal, upon us.

Both our physical and emotional health is adversely affected by stress. Because stress cannot be completely eliminated (unless we live in Hunza land) we must learn how to guard our bodies and minds against the harmful effects of stress. To reduce our vulnerability to stress the physical and psychic defenses must be worked through and released.

Stress can include excessive physical activity, family tensions, work, financial and health problems, emotional upsets and even negative attitudes and thoughts which may have a detrimental effect upon behavior and body functioning.

You may have heard that stress can cause a person to age faster than normal. And it is true. This is because of the hormonal occurrences that take place within the body when it is faced with a stress.

Stress affects the endocrine (hormone producing) system of the body largely the thyroid and the adrenals. The thyroid is a two-lobed gland about the size of a plum, located behind the Adam's apple region of the neck. The two much smaller adrenal glands are located on top of each kidney, which are located behind and underneath the lungs. The adrenals and the thyroid work closely together.

The adrenal glands provide a steady stream of sugar-raising hormones (from the adrenal cortex) which provide the fuel which the thyroid hormone uses to produce energy. It is the adrenal glands which provide extra energy when needed. For example, during stress or fear, one's "adrenals get going" releasing adrenaline (from the adrenal medulla) to provide the body with an extra boost of energy. The thyroid gland then converts this fuel into energy. To achieve maximum energy both glands must be functioning optimally.

Every time we are in a threatening or highly stressful situation, cortisol and adrenaline, glucocorticoid hormones produced by the adrenal glands, are released. This prepares the body for whatever threat is presenting itself; the heart rate increases, respiration increases, respiratory passageways dilate, digestive rate increases, speed and strength increases, etc. The effect is the same no matter what the stress; whether you are trying to run down 10 flights of stairs to get your child out of a burning building or you don't have enough money in the bank to cover the monthly bills.

## Three Major Types of Stress:

**1. Physical/Environmental:**
Toxic exposure (chemicals, etc.), light cycle disruption, allergies, temperature exposure, trauma

**2. Physiological:**
Glucose dysregulation, chronic infections, pain, lack of sleep, dietary imbalances, excessive exercise, chronic inflammation.

**3. Mental:** Anxiety, depression, alpha adrenergic stimulus

## The normal response to stress involves:

**1.** Increased adrenal corticotrophic hormone (ACTH) production

**2.** Increased cortisol & DHEA production by adrenals

**3.** Balanced Cortisol to DHEA ratio

**4.** Increased cortisol inhibits further production of adrenal hormones such as DHEA.

**5.** The increased steroid output promptly returns to normal when the stress is removed

Stress causes the increased production of chemicals known as glucocorticoid hormones. These include adrenaline and cortisol, which prepare us for "flight or fight." Continued exposure to these can cause steroid poisoning which is highly destructive to the body. Muscle wasting, fatigue, insomnia, osteoporosis, diabetes, thinning of skin, redistribution of body fat, fragility of blood vessels, hypertension, fluid retention, impaired mental function, impaired immunity and many other health related problems.

# Physiological Effects of Stress

Virtually every organ, gland and chemical constituent in the body is involved in the general stress adaptation syndrome. The adrenals response to stress has already been discussed. The kidneys regulate a steady equilibrium of the blood composition by selectively eliminating certain chemicals from the body. The liver provides energy yielding substances to meet the increased demands. It also regulates sugar concentration, protein and other important tissue foods in the blood. The liver plays a detoxifying role when there is an excess of corticoids, pollutants or poisons in the blood. White blood cells (particularly those from the thymus) regulate immune reactions to foreign substances. In addition, the brain, nerves, blood vessels, connective tissue, pituitary, and all interconnections between them are also affected by stress.

## Glucocorticoids Suppress Immune Function

High levels of glucocorticoids (such as cortisol) cause atrophy of the thymus gland, spleen, and lymph nodes, thus depressing immune responses. Glucocorticoids work with other hormones in promoting normal metabolism to make sure enough energy is provided. They increase the rate at which amino acids are removed from cells, primarily muscle cells, and transported to the liver. The amino acids may be synthesized into new proteins such as the enzymes needed for metabolic reactions. If the body's reserves of glycogen and fat are low, the liver may convert the amino acids to glucose. This conversion of a substance other than carbohydrate into glucose is called gluconeogenesis.

Glucocorticoids also help the body to store fat which explains why many people under chronic stress have weight problems.

In situations where a person cannot terminate the stress response or act it out his body administers a tiny dose of steroid poisoning. The danger of repeated inappropriate stress is much greater than any single catastrophic stress.

The human body thrives on orderliness, but the ultimate responsibility for creating order out of disorder rests with each cell.

## Stress Causes Disease and Aging

Constant or continual stress causes adaptations in the body. These first can be seen as warning signs which eventually progress to disease. Hans Selye, M.D., author of *"The Stress of Life,"* who is known as the father of the Stress Theory of Adaptation, calls this the Disease of Adaptation.

## Warning signs include:

1. General irritability, hyper-excitation or depression.
2. Pounding of the heart - an indicator of high blood pressure.
3. Dryness of the throat and mouth.
4. Impulsive behavior, emotional instability (i.e., crying).
5. Anxiety.
6. Trembling, nervous tick, nervous laughter, teeth grinding, increased smoking, hyper-mobility or other nervous behavior.
7. Insomnia.
8. Sweating.
9. Frequent need to urinate.
10. Diarrhea, indigestion, queasiness, sometimes vomiting.
11. Migraine headaches. Other aches and pains.
12. Premenstrual tension or missed periods.
13. Loss of or excessive appetite.
14. Alcohol and drug addictions.
15. Nightmares.
16. Neurotic behavior, psychoses.

The various diseases due to excessive or insufficient corticoid production associated with stress include: high blood pressure, diseases of the heart and blood vessels, diseases of the kidney, eclampsia (the gravest form of pregnancy toxicity), rheumatic and rheumatoid arthritis, inflammatory diseases of the skin and eyes, infections, allergic and hyper-sensitivity diseases, nervous and mental disease, sexual derangement, digestive diseases, metabolic diseases (such as diabetes), cancer, and diseases of resistance in general.

## Hormonal Control

Almost all animal behavior is guided by hormones including the internal integration of behavior, ranging from a simple sensory and motor reflex to feeding, mating, nest building, incubation of eggs, care of young, and migration habits. The neural and endocrine systems are so intertwined that they are sometimes viewed as one system, called the neuroendocrine system. There is a continuum between transmitters that cross the distances from one neuron to another and hormones that are carried in the blood stream with few, if any, reactions by the nervous system. Some chemicals, such as epinephrine, serve both as synaptic transmitters and glandular hormones.

The control of glucocorticoid secretion is a typical negative feedback mechanism. The two stimuli are stress and low blood level of glucocorticoids. Stress includes emotional and physical (contusions, broken bones, disease, or tissue destruction, etc.). The stress may directly stimulate the hypothalamus. For example, the hypothalamus could be stimulated by low blood pressure resulting from excessive bleeding. Or the stimulus may be related to the hypothalamus from other parts of the nervous system. In any case, either stress or an abnormally low level of glucocorticoids stimulates the hypothalamus to secrete the adreno-corticotropin hormone releasing factor (ACTHRF). This indicates the release of ACTH from the pituitary. ACTH is car-

# *Response to Stress*

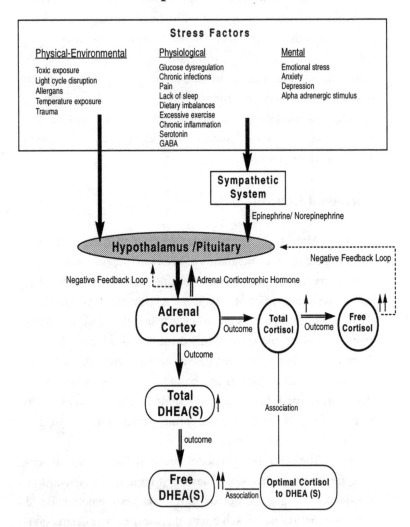

## Stress Factors

**Physical-Environmental**

Toxic exposure
Light cycle disruption
Allergans
Temperature exposure
Trauma

**Physiological**

Glucose dysregulation
Chronic infections
Pain
Lack of sleep
Dietary imbalances
Excessive exercise
Chronic inflammation
Serotonin
GABA

**Mental**

Emotional stress
Anxiety
Depression
Alpha adrenergic stimulus

**Sympathetic System**

Epinephrine/ Norepinephrine

**Hypothalamus /Pituitary**

Negative Feedback Loop

Negative Feedback Loop

Adrenal Corticotrophic Hormone

**Adrenal Cortex** — Outcome → **Total Cortisol** — Outcome → **Free Cortisol**

Outcome

**Total DHEA(S)**

outcome

Association

**Free DHEA(S)** — Association — **Optimal Cortisol to DHEA (S)**

---

### The normal response to stress involves:

- increased Adrenal Corticotrophic Hormone (ACTH)

- Increased cortisol & DHEA

- Cortisol to DHEA ratio is maintained in balance

- Increased cortisol inhibits further ACTH output thereby moderating the stress response.

- The increased steroid output promptly returns to normal when the stress is removed.

- If stress continues, a compensation occurs (see other chart for comparison)

# *Response to Chronic Stress*

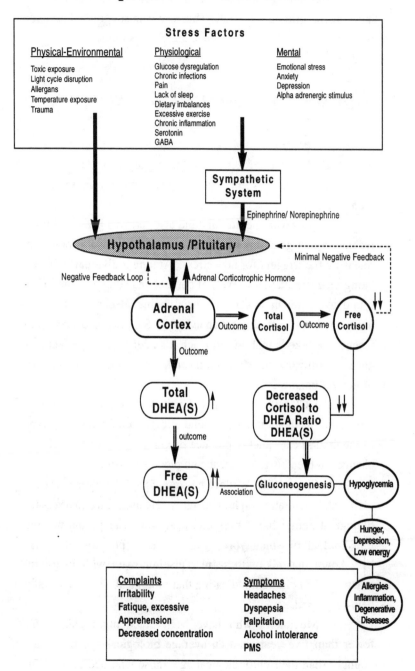

**Stress Factors**

**Physical-Environmental**

Toxic exposure
Light cycle disruption
Allergans
Temperature exposure
Trauma

**Physiological**

Glucose dysregulation
Chronic infections
Pain
Lack of sleep
Dietary imbalances
Excessive exercise
Chronic inflammation
Serotonin
GABA

**Mental**

Emotional stress
Anxiety
Depression
Alpha adrenergic stimulus

**Sympathetic System**

Epinephrine/ Norepinephrine

**Hypothalamus /Pituitary**

Minimal Negative Feedback

Negative Feedback Loop          Adrenal Corticotrophic Hormone

**Adrenal Cortex**    Outcome → **Total Cortisol**    Outcome → **Free Cortisol**

Outcome

**Total DHEA(S)**

**Decreased Cortisol to DHEA Ratio DHEA(S)**

outcome

**Free DHEA(S)**    Association    **Gluconeogenesis**    **Hypoglycemia**

**Hunger, Depression, Low energy**

**Allergies Inflammation, Degenerative Diseases**

**Complaints**
irritability
Fatigue, excessive
Apprehension
Decreased concentration

**Symptoms**
Headaches
Dyspepsia
Palpitation
Alcohol intolerance
PMS

ried through the blood to the adrenal cortex where it then stimulates glucocorticoid secretion. This results in suppressed immune
function and, among other things, increased storage of fat.

# Meditation Lowers Biological Age

The problem of how to control stress hormones is yet
unsolved. The stress reaction can be triggered in a split second
without warning. It is impossible for us to control the molecules
themselves.

However, meditation (and also, prayer) is a mind-body
technique that goes directly to the root of the stress response by
releasing the triggers for new stress. Among individuals who are
"long-term meditators," levels of cortisol and adrenaline are often
found to be much lower and their coping mechanisms almost
always tend to be stronger than average. Sickness and aging rep-
resents the body's inability to reach it's natural goal, perfect balance and fulfillment. Meditation can help the body reach its goal
of perfect balance.

UCLA physiologist R. Keith Wallace proved that tran-
scendental meditation has profound effects on the body. this type
of meditation can quickly produce deep relaxation and significant
changes in breathing, heartbeat, and blood pressure.

Since 1978, Wallace has researched the effects of tran-
scendental meditation on human aging. He used three markers for
biological aging: blood pressure, near-point vision, and hearing
threshold, all of which typically decline as people grow older. He
has shown that all of these markers improved with long-term
practice of meditation, indicating that biological age was actually
being reversed.

Meditators who have been practicing regularly for
fewer than five years had an average biological age five years
younger than their chronological age; those who had been medi-

tating longer than five years had an average biological age twelve years younger than their chronological age.

## Hormones: A Prime Marker for Aging

Levels of the most abundant hormone substance in the body, DHEA (dehydroepiandrosterone), declines in a straight line with age. Levels of DHEA peak between age 20 and 25, fall off at an increasing rate after menopause, and dwindle to 10 - 20 percent of their maximum by age 75.

DHEA is also a marker for the body's exposure to stress as its levels mirror stress as it continues to build up over a lifetime. With accelerated stress, glucocorticoids increase, lowering DHEA at the same time. On the other hand, high DHEA levels are associated with reduced incidence of coronary artery disease, breast cancer and osteoporosis. This makes sense because all these disorders of aging could be associated with excessive stress response. Higher DHEA is also associated with longer survival and decreased death from all diseases in older men.

Cortisol levels go up markedly in patients awaiting surgery; it stays up the day after surgery, with a slight elevation in DHEA. Two weeks later, cortisol is still up, but DHEA has fall-

*DHEA LEVELS DROP IN THE BODY AFTER AGE 20*

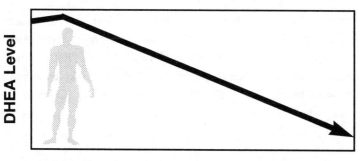

15 20 25 30 35 40 45 50 55 60 65 70 75 80 85 90

en, supporting the theory that DHEA is depleted by stress.

The logical conclusion from the evidence is that if someone can keep up their DHEA levels, their body must be resisting stress, and with fewer stress reactions, aging should be retarded.

Do those who meditate show less biological aging? Maybe. DHEA levels of experienced meditators were compared to the levels of non-meditators. The levels of DHEA were higher among meditators. Because higher DHEA levels appear in younger people, this demonstrated that meditation decreased levels of DHEA which decreased biological aging.

In other subjects, the meditating men over the age of 40 had 23 percent more DHEA, the women 47 percent more. The study states that these figures were independent of diet, exercise, alcohol consumption, and weight so these results are quite significant. The average DHEA levels of the meditators were equivalent to those of people 5 to 10 years younger.

So, what is DHEA? The rest of this book will answer this question.

## Chapter Summary

While the average life expectancy today is around age 75 the body is actually capable of living almost twice as long. The reason that most of us do not is due to the fact that we don't take care of ourselves. Aging is a part of the natural progression of life but we hasten it, creating disease and premature death.

The entire functioning of the body is regulated by hormones which circulate through our blood. Many factors, such as stress, smoking, alcohol, etc., affect hormone production disrupting homeostasis and good health. Hormone levels, DHEA in particular, serve as markers for aging and disease. DHEA levels peak between the ages of 20 and 25 and decline slowly until death.

# DHEA:
# THE MOTHER HORMONE

DHEA (dehydroepiandrosterone) is a plentiful but only vaguely understood steroid-like substance secreted by the adrenal cortex. It circulates in the bloodstream in quantities thousands of times greater than either sex hormone, estrogen and testosterone. All of the specific roles of this substance in the body are not yet conclusively known.

DHEA is structurally similar to other steroid hormones (such as estrogen, progesterone, and testosterone) but it possesses its own spectrum of biological effects. DHEA can be converted into other hormones, including estrogen, testosterone and cortisone, but it is not merely a "buffer hormone," a reservoir which the adrenals could draw upon to produce more of these other hormones. Scientists have shown that cells contain specific DHEA receptors the sole function of which is to bind DHEA. This demonstrates that DHEA is more than just a buffer hormone and that it has functions of its own in the body.

More than 90 percent of DHEA is converted to DHEA sulfate (DHEA-S) prior to circulation. DHEA-S may convert back to DHEA, convert to other hormones, or stimulate the production of other hormones by the ovaries, testes, etc. DHEA and DHEA-S are for the most part functionally interchangeable. There are some significant differences which will be noted later.

DHEA exists in the body in higher quantities than any

other hormone. Levels in the body peak around age 21 and slowly decline over the years. It is known that DHEA converts to or stimulates the production of estrogens, testosterone, progesterone, cortisone, and the many other steroid hormones as the body needs them. In a sense, DHEA, as a pre-hormone, can be called the "mother hormone." It also acts as a buffer hormone that interacts with other hormones.

DHEA is found in the brain at high concentrations. Many of its effects are related to the nervous system of which the brain is the core. This would lead us to believe that DHEA and at least some of the brain functions are closely correlated. More on this in a later chapter.

Abnormal patterns of DHEA in the body accompany and often underlie several disease states and dysfunction. These include: **Chronic Depression, Chronic Infections, Osteoporosis, AIDS, Hypoglycemia, Hypo and Hyper Adrenal Function, Stress Response, many types of Cancer, Obesity, Hypothyroidism and Alzheimer's.**

*Note the similarity of DHEA to Testosterone and Estrogen Molecules*

**DHEA Molecule**

**Estrone Molecule**

**Testosterone Molecule**

# SOME DHEA FACTS:

✚ DHEA converts to or stimulates the production of estrogens, testosterone, progesterone, cortisone, and many other steroid hormones as the body needs them.

✚ Levels of DHEA production in the body vary according to stress, fever, sudden low blood sugar, and disease states. DHEA levels are lower among smokers than among nonsmokers, and lower among heavy drinkers than among non-drinkers. Birth control pills and other synthetic hormones also deplete DHEA.

✚ Levels of salivary steroids accurately reflect fluctuating DHEA levels in the body. Salivary DHEA concentration is about 0.1 percent of its plasma concentration.

✚ In the prime of life, men produce about 31 mg DHEA daily, women, about 19 mg.

✚ DHEA has a long half-life of 8-11 hours due to its slow clearance by the liver and kidney.

✚ DHEA is found in the brain in very high concentrations equal to that in the adrenal cortex.

✚ Abnormal patterns of DHEA accompany and often underlie several disease states and dysfunction.

✚ Supplements include **DHEA-S**, which requires a prescription, and **free form DHEA** which is available over the counter in tablet, capsule, transdermal, sublingual and spray delivery systems.

# ADRENAL HORMONE SYNTHESIS

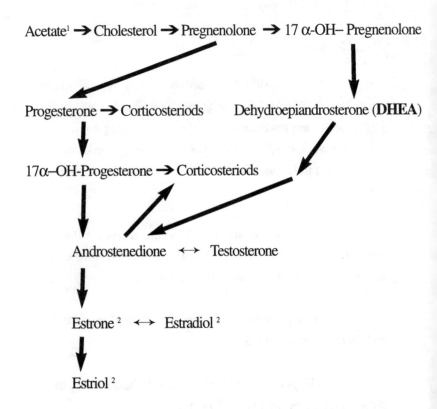

Acetate[1] → Cholesterol → Pregnenolone → 17 α-OH– Pregnenolone

Progesterone → Corticosteriods     Dehydroepiandrosterone (**DHEA**)

17α–OH-Progesterone → Corticosteriods

Androstenedione ↔ Testosterone

Estrone[2] ↔ Estradiol[2]

Estriol[2]

**NOTE 1:** *Acetate is obtained from metabolism of sugar and fatty acids.*

**NOTE 2:** *Estrone, Estradiol and Estriol are forms of Estrogen.*

# DHEA Provides Alternative Pathway

DHEA is the precursor of some 10 different steroidal hormones associated with youth. We all know that with increasing age women suffer from decreased estrogen production and men from decreased testosterone production. Hormone replacement therapy providing synthetic estrogen to women and synthetic testosterone to men seems to help alleviate some of the problems associated with aging. Because there are so many different hormones circulating about the body supplementation of just one or two hormones causes an imbalance and side effects occur.

While estrogen has shown to have beneficial cardiovascular effects progestins exert a detrimental effect on blood lipids by increasing LDL and reducing HDL cholesterol. Without progestin prolonged estrogen therapy increases the risk of endometrial cancer. In summary, balance of all circulating hormones is the key. In the long run, imbalance promotes sickness and aging.

DHEA provides an alternative pathway to the gonadal hormones such as testosterone, estrogens and also cortisone. It is necessary for at least 18 different steroidal hormones. It is self regulating. Only those hormones needed are produced.

By looking at the flow chart you can see that when progesterone is deficient hormone synthesis can be achieved through the alternative DHEA pathway.

In addition to its precursor function in the formation of testosterone and estrogens supplemental DHEA has been shown to lessen many age related symptoms in both human and animal studies and it dramatically extends life spans of rodents. This may be in part due to its effects on hormone synthesis but DHEA also has additional biologic properties.

DHEA is under close scrutiny as an anti-obesity treatment in women and for its anti-cancer influences.

# Pregnenolone is Precursor to DHEA

Pregnenolone, a hormone also produced from choles-
terol in our adrenal glands (and also liver, skin, testicles, ovaries
and brain) is the biological precursor to DHEA. As the "grand-
mother" to all steroid hormones, pregnenolone is known as the
hormone balancer and has the special ability to increase the levels of steroid hormones which are deficient in our bodies and to
reduce the levels of excess circulating hormones. As a steriod hormone precursor, it is believed that pregnenolone is involved in
every biochemical action inhibited by any steriod hormone. The
potential of involvement is very wide and may impact memory,
mental alertness, stress responses, female and male reproduction,
immunity, joint and tissue function, inflammation and more. It is
also believed that pregnenolone is highly discriminative as it converts to other hormones only as they are needed by the body. This
reduces the risk for side effects which is sometimes experienced
with DHEA capsules when taken in excess.

# DHEA: Biologic and Clinical Action

In the body, DHEA has action through the steroids it
creates and also directly through its own cellular receptors.

DHEA affects the entire endocrine system by regulation through enzyme inhibition or activation. This means, it can
stimulate the production of other hormones, of most significance,
estrogen by the ovaries and testosterone by the testicles.

DHEA has demonstrated broad beneficial potential in
many detailed studies on prevention of carcinogenesis, tumor
growth, radiation, skin, hair, aging, prolactin, pregnancy, hypertension, thyroid function, bone growth, and effects on CNS
behavior and response.

## Anti-Aging Effects of DHEA

DHEA is rapidly becoming known as the anti-aging miracle of the 21st Century. It reaches its highest concentration during puberty and declines as the body ages. It is necessary for at least 18 different steroidal hormones associated with youth. These include estrogen, progesterone, cortisone, and testosterone. Levels of these hormones decline with age. Studies show that testosterone (synthetic, of course) injected into males, can actually dramatically decrease biological age, decreasing many of the symptoms of aging. The same is true for women and estrogen. Thus, Hormone Replacement Therapy was conceived. Even better, the introduction of DHEA.

Great excitement was generated in the late 1980's when Dr. Arthur Schwartz, a biochemist at Temple University, administered DHEA to mice and observed a remarkable reversal of aging: Old mice regained youthful vigor, and their coats resumed their former sleek and glossy texture; incipient cancers, whether naturally occurring or induced by artificial means, disappeared; obese animals returned to normal weight; immune response increases; and animals with diabetes improved drastically. The race to patent a version of the DHEA molecule began, although, the original substances were patented in Germany in the early 1900's.

## DHEA Has Multiple Effects on the Body

DHEA is converted into other hormones by the body and therefore acts as a precursor or a pro-hormone. DHEA has been called a "buffer hormone" that interacts with other hormones. DHEA gives rise to the sex steroids as well as additional hormones which have a wide variety of physiologic functions. If the levels of a particular sex hormone are low, DHEA can stimulate its production through either the appropriate gland (ovaries or testes) or through biosynthesis.

The varied action of this hormone is based upon the particular physiologic setting of the individual. DHEA appears to work in widely divergent systems against a variety of targets, depending on the state of the host.

DHEA regulates diabetes, obesity, carcinogenesis, tumor growth, virus and bacterial infection, stress, pregnancy, hypertension, collagen and skin integrity, fatigue, depression, memory and immune responses.

### The known actions of DHEA include:

Regulates hormones through specific or non-specific hormone receptors.

Inhibits an antiproliferative enzyme, G-6-PD.

Increases fat metabolism through thermogenesis.

Decreases desire to eat, possibly through its effects on insulin.

Decreases negative effects of stress.

Stimulates T-lymphocytes / Enhances interleukin 2 production.

Anti-osteoporosis / Improves calcium absorption.

Anti-inflammatory.

These will be explained in more detail later.

# Production of DHEA

Adrenal corticotropic hormones (ACTH) and other non ACTH regulatory components control adrenal steroid secretion. External factors such as stress and illness play significant roles in determining output (57 percent reduction in DHEA levels following ACTH stimulus due to chronic stress, 77 percent reduction due to chronic illness).

**The following internal factors play a role in DHEA production:**

**Genetics:** About 65 percent of production is related to heredity.

**24-hour Circadian Variation:** Account for daily fluctuations of 13 percent.

**Seasonal Circadian Variation:** An increase in plasma concentration of DHEA can be seen during the winter months.

**Age:** Levels of DHEA production increase through puberty, peaking between age 20 and 25. After this time production slowly diminishes. Lower levels of production decreases health and lower levels are associated with dysfunction including:

> Psychosomatic Disorders
> Chronic Fatigue Syndrome
> Stress Induced Disease
> Chronic Depression
> Reduced Immunity
> Chronic Infections
> Osteoporosis
> Hypoglycemia
> Diabetes
> Stress Response
> Hypothyroidism
> Alzheimer's
> AIDS

Alzheimer's patients have 46 percent lower levels of DHEA than age-matched controls and have an elevated level of cortisol. Elevations of cortisol levels are shown to be damaging in animal studies. DHEA administration is known to improve memory function in aging animals.

DHEA levels were significantly elevated in men who

had survived heart attacks at least five months earlier. Men with at least 50 percent coronary blockage on angiography, but with no heart attacks, had normal DHEA values. DHEA levels may be a marker for underlying protective effects or be a protective substance itself.

*Note:* Individuals who suffer from chronic elevated ACTH and hypercortisol with Cushing's disease do not experience increased DHEA levels.

# Effects of Stress on DHEA

**Exercise:** Strenuous exercise such as running, swimming, football, weight lifting, etc. increases serum concentrations of cortisol and DHEA in both men and women. In contrast, marathon runners (1100 Km for 20 days) show no change in DHEA and a return to normal cortisol levels after completion of a 24-40-week training program.

**Hypertension:** DHEA excretion rates through the urine were significantly decreased by 85-95 percent below controls in clinically hypertensive patients. Further investigation revealed that circulating DHEA levels were not different in hypertensive individuals when compared to their age matched control.

**Emotional Stress:** Stressful events such as anticipated death or surgery of a family member, hospital admission, public speaking, mental performance testing, residence relocation in the elderly, depress DHEA production. The Cortisol/DHEA ratio in individuals with panic disorder is depressed by about 50 percent.
**Obesity:** The cortisol secretion rate is increased in obese individuals. Production rates of DHEA are higher than normal in obese individuals. However, circulating DHEA levels remain

unchanged due to an accelerated metabolic clearance rate.

Diversion of the precursors for both cortisol and adrenal andro-gens reduces DHEA output. This may be due to nutritional fac-tors, stress, illness, chemical alteration through drugs, etc. Cholesterol is one of the precursors for DHEA.

**Diet:** Vegetarian diets and the intake of saturated and unsaturat-ed fats do not significantly affect DHEA levels. However, decreases in other steroids such as androstenedione, extrone and estradiol have been reported.

**Drugs:** A number of drugs, not only pharmaceuticals, but also alcohol and tobacco, lower levels of DHEA, probably due to the increased stress on the body. Intake of synthetic steroid hor-mones also lowers DHEA levels. Birth control pills especially have a detrimental effect.

# Alcohol Lowers Levels of DHEA and Other Hormones

Alcohol puts an added stress on the body. There is a significant amount of research that shows the detrimental effects of alcohol to the many hormones in the body, including DHEA.

Women who are heavy drinkers have been found to have a DHEA-S level 39 percent lower than non drinking con-trols. In addition, testosterone levels were 65 percent higher, and progesterone levels were 23 percent lower. (Valimaki)

Alcohol is known to decrease production of proges-terone, specifically during the critical time of pregnancy and is believed to be a cause of the numerous associated problems. (Ahluwalia)

Excessive drinking is also known to decrease thyroid hormone production. (Jimenez)

## Effects of Alcohol on Men

Numerous studies of men drinkers show a significant reduction in serum testosterone. (Sengupta )

There is also an abundance of evidence for the adverse effects of chronic alcoholism on serum hormones and sperm count. These may be responsible for the fertility disorders common in chronic alcoholics: (Gomathi and Farinati)

Marked reduction in sperm concentration

Increase in the number of abnormal sperm

Testosterone  levels decrease

Oestradiol  (estrogen) levels  increase

## Effects of Alcohol on Women

Alcohol induces a number of sex hormone disturbances in women. In premenopausal females alcohol consumption increases the frequency of menstrual disturbances, abortions, miscarriages, and infertility.

Chronic alcohol abuse leads to reduced concentrations of  steroids, and these changes may be seen before severe liver dysfunction has appeared. In women liver dysfunction leads to earlier occurrence of menopause in comparison with normal controls, while information is insufficient or lacking regarding the influence upon fertility, pregnancy outcome and sexual behavior in women. (Becker)

In women, the estradiol to testosterone ratio was significantly lower in patients with HCC than in controls with cirrhosis. (Farinati)

## Alcohol Has Negative Effects During Pregnancy

Alcohol consumption changes the hormone secretory

responses induced by epidermal growth factor in choriocarcinoma cells. Clinical data have implicated alcohol as an embryotoxic agent that disrupts normal placental structure and function and could potentially explain the reasoning behind alcohol toxicity during pregnancy. (Wimalasena)

## Alcohol Lowers Levels of Growth Hormone

Alcohol-dependent patients showed significantly less Growth Hormone secretion in all neuroendocrine tests than non-drinkers. (Dettling)

## Alcohol Lowers Levels of DHEA and Progesterone

A study published earlier this year at the University of Helsinki, in Finland revealed that women who were heavy drinkers (but did not have liver disease) had the following blood levels compared to non-drinking control women: (Valimaki)

Testosterone was 65% higher.

Progesterone level was 23% lower.

DHEA-S level was 39% lower.

## Alcohol Spurs Early Onset of Menopause

In a study at the University of Copenhagen, Denmark, Becker and associates examined the average age for onset of menopause and sex hormones in postmenopausal women with alcoholic and non-alcoholic liver disease. They found that all patients were significantly younger at the time of natural menopause compared to non-drinking controls. (Becker)

They also found that compared to controls, non-cirrhotic alcoholic women had significantly reduced levels of DHEA-S, significantly more alcoholic cirrhotic women had detectable estrogen (oestradiol), elevated concentrations of estrogen (oestrone) and sex hormone binding globulin (SHBG) and reduced levels testosterone,

Women with non-alcoholic cirrhosis had significantly

41

elevated concentrations of sex hormone binding globulin and reduced sulphate, testosterone, androstenedione (which converts to the estrogen and testosterone sex hormones) and DHEA-S. (Becker)

## Social Drinking Has Major Influence on Hormone Levels of Postmenopausal Women

Dr. J. S. Gavaler, University of Pittsburgh, Pennsylvania, conducted a trial to investigate the effects of social drinking (moderate alcoholic beverage consumption) on the hormonal status of postmenopausal women. The results revealed that moderate alcohol intake exerts a major influence not only on estradiol and testosterone, but also on the estrogen-responsive pituitary hormones.

The hormonal status of postmenopausal women with alcohol-induced cirrhosis was compared with normal alcohol-abstaining control women. There are significant differences in levels of all hormones; furthermore, hormonal interrelationships are also disrupted. Of major interest also is that the degree of hormone level abnormality is related to the severity of liver disease. (Gavaler)

# Chapter Summary

DHEA is produced and secreted by the adrenal glands. There is more DHEA circulating in the body than any other hormone. DHEA converts to or stimulates the production of estrogens, testosterone, progesterone, cortisone, and many other steroid hormones as the body needs them. It therefore is referred to as "The Mother Hormone." A number of factors can alter the amount of DHEA produced and ultimately affect the levels of these other hormones as well. Stress is a major factor contributing to our levels of DHEA production. DHEA has a number of direct and indirect beneficial metabolic effects on the body.

# DHEA: THERAPEUTIC EFFECTS

Until recently, DHEA research has focused on its place as an intermediate in sex steroid synthesis. Just in the last decade, DHEA has been found to have numerous properties on its own. DHEA can prevent cardiogenesis and slow the development of diabetes. Interest is rapidly growing in DHEA's relationship to atherosclerosis, hypertension, memory disorders, fat mobilization and cancer prevention and treatment. Clinical trials are in progress in the area of cancer, diabetes, obesity, osteoporosis, hypercholesterolemia, Alzheimer's Disease, AIDS, Lupus, and multiple sclerosis.

DHEA is a potent inhibitor of glucose-6-phosphate dehydrogenase, the enzyme necessary for cancer cell proliferation.

In man, serum levels of DHEA peak in early adulthood and drop markedly with age. Epidemiologic evidence indicates that these low levels of DHEA are linked to an increased risk of developing cancer or of death from cardiovascular disease. Like cancer, atherosclerosis is a proliferative process characterized by both initiation and promotion phases.

DHEA has also shown to increase resistance to viral or bacterial infection.

DHEA has been thought to act as a naturally-occurring digitalis. Digitalis strengthens the heart muscle contractions and is used to treat heart failure.

The clinical experience with DHEA suggest it may be useful in fatigue syndromes and in lowering blood cholesterol.

**NOTE:** To date, almost all of the published research conducted on DHEA has been done with free form DHEA or DHEA-S. Very little published research has been done on naturally derived extracts from wild yams.

There are some side effects which accompany synthetic DHEA supplementation in some specific conditions, but to a much lesser extent compared to those occurring with synthetic hormone analogs.

Naturally-derived hormones, such as progesterone from wild yam extract, seem to have much less risk of side effects compared to synthetic progesterone analogs. This will be detailed later in this book.

## DHEA and Safety

DHEA has wide past clinical experience and is remarkably free of side effects when taken in the proper amount, especially when compared to conventional treatments. Signals that your supplemental DHEA intake may be too high include the following:

**Acne**

**Facial hair (women)**

**Rapid heart beat**

**Irritability/ Anxiety**

**Headaches**

**Difficulty sleeping**

If you experience any of these while taking DHEA you should reduce your intake. For optimal results, contact a health-care practitioner familiar with DHEA who can monitor your blood levels. Remember, women need less than men and the healthier and younger you are the less you need because your body may still be producing adequate amounts.

Current DHEA clinical research is focused on the prevention or treatment of cancer and atherosclerosis. However, it has much broader potential: DHEA has been found to be useful in the treatment of patients with Alzheimer's and other memory disorders, osteoporosis. DHEA actually restores bone density, diabetes, fat metabolism, weight problems, hypertension, multiple sclerosis, angioneurotic edema, and arthritis, cirrhosis, and psoriasis because of the immunostimulating anti-inflammatory action of DHEA.

The beneficial effects of DHEA supplementation for women are especially encouraging. Hormone therapy with synthetic progesterone (or progestins) and synthetic estrogen (which is made from the urine of pregnant horses) is widely prescribed for menopausal therapy in spite of all of the known side effects and risks associated with taking them. Synthetic progesterone is associated with an increased risk of uterine and breast cancer, blood clots, fluid retention (swelling), breast tenderness, weight gain, depression, skin breakouts, alopecia (hair loss), masculizing effects (i.e., excess body hair), insomnia, amenorrhea, rise in blood pressure, migraine headaches, and an increase in LDL and reduced HDL cholesterol levels. Estrogen therapy increases the risk of endometrial cancer.

## DHEA Calms Hyperproduction Actions

One of the most interesting aspects of supplemental DHEA is its ability to suppress overactive body processes termed "hyperproductive syndrome." This includes over-production of nucleic acids, fats, hormones, and cells which may be considered cancerous. This also may apply to autoimmune conditions such as rheumatoid arthritis and lupus, where the body attacks its own healthy tissue.

DHEA is responsible for a decline in a number of degenerative diseases through its effects against this hyperproductive syndrome. DHEA inhibits enzyme systems necessary for building new cells, i.e., nucleic acids, lipids and steroids. With the age related decline in DHEA levels proliferative or degenerative events develop related to the loss of DHEA as a key regulatory hormone controlling key enzymes. Under appropriate circumstances, i.e., carcinogenesis, obesity, diabetes and stress, DHEA functions as an "anti-hormone."

The late Dr. Norman Applezweig, a New York biochemist, suggested that DHEA "cannot serve to 'excite' in the true classical sense of hormone action, but that it acts to 'de-excite' metabolic processes which overproduce when high DHEA is in short supply."

Dr. Applezweig believed that unlike hormones that excite cells in activity DHEA "de-excites" the body's process. Some of the diseases of aging are caused by the runaway production of nucleic acids, fats, and hormones. DHEA slows down their production and thereby slows down aging. The pituitary gland produces releasing hormones, which stimulate testes, ovaries, and the adrenal glands, to produce steroid hormones. These steroid hormones circulate through the bloodstream to the hypothalamus in the brain which sends a feedback signal to the pituitary gland saying "make more" or "make less." With natural DHEA, the pituitary gland will continue to produce steroid hormones. The pituitary gland stops producing when anabolic steroids are taken.

Whatever its mechanism of physiologic action DHEA is perhaps our most significant endocrine biomarker that declines with age.

It is not yet understood if the age-related decrease is pertinent to the pathology or functional changes seen in aging and if the anti-carcinogenesis or anti-diabetogenic action of DHEA has relevance to any of the above. DHEA has an apparent effect on improving clinical fatigue, mobilizing fat, lowering cholesterol levels, and preventing arteriosclerosis.

## Osteoporosis

DHEA has demonstrated improved intestinal calcium absorption possibly due to its effects on vitamin D metabolism. Studies also show the relationship between adrenal steroids and reduction of osteoporotic bone loss.

## Immune System

DHEA has a direct stimulating effect on white blood cells called T-lymphocytes in-vivo and in-vitro by enhancing interleukin-2 (IL-2) production in cell-mediated immune responses. Additionally, DHEA can overcome the immuno-suppressive effect of cortisol on T-lymphocytes. Cortisol (resulting from high stress) depresses IL-2 production causing T-cell levels to drop.

## Blood Lipids

Clinical studies show that supplemental oral DHEA-S intake can lower total serum cholesterol, particularly LDL (low density lipoprotein) cholesterol, by an average of 18 percent. The decrease in total cholesterol occurs without changing food intake, activity level, or body weight

## Weight

High doses of supplemental DHEA-S (1,500 mg/day, oral) given to healthy males for one month caused a 31 percent reduction in body fat content without changes in dieting or exercise. Total weight did not change significantly indicating an increase in lean muscle weight.

CAUTION: Doses this high may cause harm to your liver and are not recommended unless you are under the close supervision of a physician who is familiar with the use of DHEA for such purpose. Lower levels around 25-50mg for women and 25-100mg for men still have a safe and beneficial effect on weight.

DHEA encourages normal body composition. Supplemental DHEA has shown to encourage weight loss in those who are overweight and encourage weight gain in underweight individuals.

One study showed that removal of the adrenal gland slowed weight gain in young obese mice, demonstrating the importance of the adrenal hormones such as DHEA for proper weight maintenance.

# Anti-Aging

DHEA is rapidly becoming known as the anti-aging miracle of the 20th Century. It reaches its highest concentration during puberty and declines as the body ages. It is necessary for at least 18 different steroidal hormones associated with youth, including estrogen, progesterone, cortisone, and testosterone. Levels of all of these hormones decline with age.

The various hormonal effects of DHEA appear to decrease bone reabsorption and increase bone formation.

Scientists presently are experimenting with supplemental DHEA to confirm earlier studies that demonstrate an ability to improve memory, improve sex drive, prevent conditions associated with increased age such as cancer, Alzheimer's disease, multiple sclerosis and memory loss.

We must also ask why DHEA is found in the brain in such large quantities and how this might have relevance to memory, mood, neuroendocrine changes, neuro-immunomodulation, and neurite formation?

# DHEA Converts to Estrogens and Testosterone

Supplemental DHEA given orally has proven to be highly beneficial. Healthy women given DHEA rapidly convert it to estrogens causing a 300-500 percent temporary increase in levels. Testosterone levels also temporarily increased by 300-400 percent. These effects occur only if the body naturally requires such a conversion. Therefore, a supplemental DHEA is non-toxic and far safer than taking synthetic hormone or steroid analogs.

Enhanced immune functions means enhanced protection against viral infections ranging from the common cold to herpes. Further, it means revitalization of all bodily functions including sexual health and slowing of the aging process.

# DHEA Levels Decline with Age

The decline in DHEA levels in the body as we grow older is widely recognized. At age 60 or 70, blood levels are only 10-20 percent of what they were at age 20. Estrogen and testosterone levels are lower. Requirements for stress hormones may be slightly less than they were when in our 20's and 30's, but stress and other influences throughout life dwindle any DHEA in reserve.

In young females, the ovaries are responsible for 50 percent of androstenedione (which converts to the estrogen and testosterone sex hormones), with the remainder coming from the conversion of DHEA. With aging, the ovary, despite estrogen loss, is still able to synthesize androstenedione and testosterone.

However, clinical estrogen substitution does nothing to restore DHEA levels, suggesting a non-estrogen dependent role for ovarian function in regulating DHEA production. Studies have demonstrated that removal of the ovaries has a significant influence on DHEA levels enhancing the age-related decline.

DHEA decline is probably an indication of unhealthy changes in the adrenals. This suggests that we must look at other androgens whose levels are fairly stable despite aging as they may have more physiologic importance to the maintenance of youthful survival which may go beyond their role as sex steroids.

Aging, as related to high insulin levels, may provide insight into DHEA's functional role for preventing obesity, insulin resistance, and hyperphagia in rodents. It is the clinical decline in DHEA induced by insulin and suggests that age-related decline in DHEA may be a function of increased age-related insulin production.

However, there seems to be an opposing action between DHEA and testosterone on insulin resistance. If this is so, aging would result in hypothalamic damage resulting in hypersecretion of insulin and glucagon. Hyper-insulinemia, insulin resistance and hyperglycemia play a causative pathologic role in senescence. This is an extension of the concept of the age-related hyperproductive syndrome due to the decline in DHEA.

As an anti-aging hormone, we have to consider the potential of DHEA as a stress-modulating steroid. It is suggested that DHEA has an adrenocortical stress-mediated blocking action. Low concentrations of DHEA to cortisol with age can lead to age-related stress induced CNS injury.

The anti-diabetogenic action of DHEA may also relate to DHEA's action in blocking corticosteroid responses. In this regard, aging has been likened to a cushingoid response, that leads to age related diabetes and degenerative disease which may be impeded by DHEA.

DHEA levels are low in intensive care patients who also show a reduction in DHEA/cortisol ratios although ACTH responses can be normal. (Wade)

Cortisol levels rise in severe illness, in burn patients and in both alcoholic and non alcoholic livers, at the expense of other steroids. There is a significant fall in DHEA. Patients with anorexia nervosa have disassociation between adrenal androgens and cortisol with low levels of DHEA. With exercise, DHEA levels rise along with other androgens.

# DHEA Dosages

Although DHEA is a steroid it does not seem to exhibit the strong hormone influences of "fully formed" steroids like estrogen, testosterone, or progesterone. As a consequence, this steroid "precursor" possess a minimal anabolic, androgenic and estrogenic activity.

Ideal supplemental DHEA dosage can vary dramatically from person to person. Age is a strong factor, but other biological influences may be significant. DHEA dosages range from 5-500 mg. Before and after tests of blood DHEA may be recommended to assess the dose.

Anti-aging doses would be quite low, taking only enough to raise the levels to a normal 20 year old, which would be approximately 31 mg in men, 19 mg in women. Because men naturally manufacture higher amounts than women do, men can take higher supplemental amounts.

Actual assimilation of capsules is only about 50% in healthy individuals. This means a 50 mg capsule could probably increase your DHEA level by about 25 mg. As you can see, this is too much for many women (who are healthy) and may be too much for men who are still producing a fair amount on their own. Older and individuals with certain health problems may have as assimilation factor of less than 50%.

Long-term preventative "anti-aging" DHEA supplementation of 5 to 50 mg daily is perfectly safe because this amount simply restores the level the body had when it was producing at our optimum level.

Therapeutic doses may be much higher, beginning around 200 mg. Some studies have been done using as much as

1,600 mg daily, while it is important to realize that no long term human studies have been done to show this is a safe level. Laboratory animals given very high doses for prolonged periods showed evidence of liver damage. (Schwartz)

Some physicians who prescribe 100 mg dosages recommend cycling, taking DHEA daily for 4 weeks, then taking 2 to 4 weeks off, before starting the next cycle. This is to protect the adrenal glands and promote continued optimal production.

As with other steroid hormones, it is recommended that intake levels begin low and gradually increase to the proper dose. If taking high doses (over 100 mg daily), one should not suddenly stop, but slowly decrease the dosage to "wean" yourself off.

If you do experience side effects, such as acne, unwanted hair growth, headaches, sleeplessness, fatigue, and in some cases, irritability and rapid heart beat, the amount you are taking may be too high and you should reduce the dosage immediately to reduce stress on the body. You want the DHEA to help you deal with stress, not to take too much so it *causes* stress!

If you are unsure about how much DHEA to take for your individual situation, it is strongly recommended that you see a physician so that blood levels can be monitored. DHEA levels are measured in nanograms per deciliter of blood. Acceptable levels for men is above 750 ng/dL, for women, above 550 ng/dL. Supplementation may be recommended for levels below these figures. (*see next page*)

No human studies have demonstrated any harmful side effects of DHEA at low "anti-aging" maintenance doses under 50 mg daily for men or women. Laboratory animals given very, very high doses for prolonged periods showed evidence of liver damage. (Schwartz) Remember that almost any substance, even water, can be dangerous if abused or used improperly. DHEA is nothing to be afraid of as long as you are taking the correct amount.

It is usually suggested that you take your DHEA supplement in the morning upon arising. This is when DHEA in the body is naturally at its highest level. Because free form DHEA has a shorter half-life in the body compared to the compound DHEA-S, you may wish to split the dosage taking half in the morning and half in the evening to maintain an even blood level throughout each 24 hour period.

## *Chapter Summary*

This chapter summarizes the various therapeutic benefits of DHEA. DHEA has shown to have positive effects against cancer, diabetes, obesity, osteoporosis, hypercholesterolemia, heart disease, Alzheimer's disease, memory loss, AIDS, lupus, arthritis, and multiple sclerosis. In most cases the goal to replenish your levels to what they were when they were naturally highest. This maintenance anti-aging doses would probably be between 5 and 50 mg daily while therapeutic doses may be as high as 500 mg daily. It is recommended that DHEA be used under the supervision of a physician to ensure proper intake levels and to prevent or reduce the risk of side effects.

# DHEA AND IMMUNITY

Immune function normally declines with advancing age leading to decreased ability to fight off infections and illness.

The relationship between DHEA and the immune system may be the most significant of all. DHEA has shown to enhance our immunity in a variety of ways against a number of degenerative and infectious disease conditions. DHEA is believed to stimulate T-cells, B-cells, and macrophages by interfering with glucocorticoid immuno-suppression. DHEA protects against both bacterial and viral infections. Some of these include the deadly enterovirus and other herpes virus infections.

Although most major adrenocortical hormones, such as cortisone, cause immune suppression, DHEA has prevented death from infection with two different types of viruses and a fatal streptococcus infection. Scientists believe that DHEA does not necessarily affect the virus itself, but it strengthens one's immune resistance to infection. (Ben-Nathan)

## Anti-Stress Effects of DHEA

One of the most common comments among individuals supplementing DHEA is that they feel more relaxed and less stressed, with an increased ability to deal with day-to-day activities.

Studies show that DHEA has demonstrated anti-stress effects by enhancing immunity. When rats were inoculated with a virulent West Nile Virus and then subjected to the stress of immersion in cold water, 67 percent of them died. However, animals treated with DHEA prior to inoculation had a significantly reduced mortality rate demonstrating DHEA's anti-stress effects.

Enhanced immune functions means enhanced protection against viral infections ranging from the common cold to herpes. Further, it means revitalization of all bodily functions, including sexual health, and slowing of the aging process.

### DHEA Aids Healing Following Burn Injury

Healing of the skin following thermal injury is aided by postburn subcutaneous administration of DHEA. Clinical trials demonstrate that postburn intervention with DHEA, either directly or indirectly, maintained a normal architecture in most of the dermal capillaries within burn-exposed tissue. These findings suggest that systemic intervention therapy of burn patients with DHEA is useful in preventing the progressive tissue destruction caused by poor blood flow commonly associated with burns. (Araneo)

# DHEA Enhances Immune Activity

Overall immune function is known to decline with age and declining DHEA levels. As immune function declines there is increased incidence of infection, cancer, and autoimmune conditions. Immunologic competence is largely dependent on both the ability and speed of response to antigens by specific cellular elements. In a study led by Dr. Samuel Yen, nine healthy elderly men (mean age, 63) took 50 mg. encapsulated DHEA orally for 20 weeks. At this time their immune levels were checked and compared with their pre-DHEA baseline levels. The results showed that DHEA significantly enhanced immune functioning. There were no adverse effects in any of the individuals participating in the study. The researchers noted that the increase in bioavailable IGF-1 could help to explain the effects because of the possible mitogenic effects on immune cell function. (Khorram, Yen, et al)

  This study indicates that DHEA may play an important role in immuno-deficient states, including aging itself.

## DHEA Effects at 20 Weeks

(unless otherwise indicated)

**IGF-1 levels**
 (insulin-glucose factor 1)  Increased 20%

**IFG-1/GFBP-1**  Increased 32%

**Monocytes**  Increased 45% (2 wks)
        Increased 35%

**B cell population**  Increased 35% (2 wks)
        Increased 29% (10 wks)

**B cell** mitogenic response without
changes in serum IgG, IgA & IgM Increased 62% (12 wks)

**T cell mitogenic response**  Increased 40%

**IL-2R (CD25+)**  Increased 39%

**Serum sIL-2R** (suggest functional
T-lymphocyte activation)  Increased 20% (12-20 wks)

**In-vitro mitogen-stimulated
release of IL-2 & IL-6**  Increased 50% & 30%,
        respectively

**NK cell number**  Increased 22-37%

**Concomitant cytoxity**  Increased 45%

# DHEA Increases Effectiveness of Vaccines

As we grow older, the immune system weakens to such an extent that vaccinations do little good. But when old-age mice were given DHEA-S, their immune systems were suddenly and completely rejuvenated. In addition, other signs of old age began to fall away. They started gaining weight instead of losing it. Their energy and vitality were greatly improved. *"Even with quite low levels of DHEA-S, mouse immune systems aged backward for a year. And the mice given DHEA-S invariably outlived mice that were not given the hormone. After two years, we sometimes had only five out of twenty control animals left, but nearly all ten of the mice on DHEA-S were still alive."* (Daynes)

Other studies have shown similar immune dysfunction reversal with DHEA. (Araneo) The antibody response of mice to a vaccine was found to decline with age at Kentucky University's Sanders-Brown Center on Aging. DHEA significantly enhanced splenic immune responses and the discrepancy reversed. (Garg)

# Thymus Gland Protection

The thymus gland, located behind the breastbone, regulates T-cells, the immune system's principal "detectives" and "killers." The thymus control what and when the T-cells attack and control other white blood cells that make antibodies. When the thymus gland no longer works efficiently, bacteria, viruses, cancer cells, and other harmful substances are not attacked but are left free to invade body tissues.

Sometimes directions from the thymus are so confusing that some of the body's own cells attack the body itself, creating autoimmune conditions such as arthritis, lupus, and multiple sclerosis. As the immune function declines, the shrinkage and incapacitation of the thymus gland is associated with increased susceptibility to bacterial infections, viral infections, cancers, and other types of diseases.

**DHEA Slows Shrinkage of the Thymus**

DHEA protects thymic function by slowing shrinkage of the gland. In one controlled study, the normal damaging immuno-suppressive impact dexamethasone, a synthetic gluco-corticoid, was significantly and successfully slowed by DHEA. Compared with controls, those who receive pretreatment with DHEA also resulted in significantly lessened dexamethasone induced thymic atrophy. (Blauer)

In another study, the thymus gland showed improved regulatory control over the functional capabilities of mature recirculating T-cells when repotentiated by DHEA. (Wiedmeier) Some clinicians believe DHEA can actually regenerate the thymus gland in humans.

# Autoimmune Diseases

Conditions in which the immune system mistakenly attacks the body's own tissues are called autoimmune diseases. Various types of arthritis, lupus, inflammatory bowel disease (ulcerative colitis and Crohn's disease), and other inflammatory or connective tissue disorders are considered autoimmune diseases. Many other conditions, including allergies, asthma, diabetes, hypertension, and heart disease, are also thought to be autoimmune related.

# Lupus

Studies in animals suggest that DHEA may have a beneficial effect on the process of autoimmune attack. The New Zealand Black Mouse is a strain of mice that spontaneously develops an autoimmune syndrome resembling lupus. Administering DHEA to these animals prevented the kidney failure and hemolytic anemia associated with this syndrome.

Excellent results were seen among women with systemic lupus erythematosus (SLE) in a recent double-blind, placebo-controlled clinical trial with 200 mg DHEA for three months. The women taking the DHEA experienced fewer lupus flares, their overall disease activity improved, and they were able to decrease their dosage of prednisone compared to the placebo group, The women were pleased with the results of taking the DHEA in spite of the mild acne that some of the women experienced. (The study results were published in the December 1995, *Arthritis and Rheumatism*, Vol 38; No.12, pg 1826-1831. Ronald Vollenhoven, et. al)

        I have spoken to individuals suffering from lupus who are also successfully using 200 mg DHEA daily. Jeannie M. of Los Angeles, C.A., "swears by it" exclaiming that nothing can stop the pain of an attack like DHEA. She states that an attack can bring about incredible disabling pain, where she is unable to move, but with DHEA, she can return to normal within 30 minutes. She reports she has also found DHEA to help with blood sugar regulation and to help with fainting spells, reduce night sweats, reduce mouth sores and increase her energy level tremendously. She states she doesn't want to be without it and carries it with her where ever she goes.

        The Lupus Foundation of America (1-800-558-1021) in Washington, D.C., is reportedly currently investigating the effects of DHEA and Lupus. They plan to make their findings public when the investigation is complete.

## DHEA and Regulation of Interleukin-2 Production

        DHEA has been shown to increase the production of interleukin-2, a component of the immune system, which is consistently decreased in individuals with lupus. The immune system's T-cells contain a specific DHEA receptor. DHEA is, thus, believed to regulate the production of interleukin-2 and this may be yet another mechanism by which it improves immune function. (Meikle) The drug-induced suppression of T-cells, B-cells, and antibody production in rats were all reversed after administration of DHEA. (Rasmussen)

Burned mice were able to maintain normal immune function when DHEA was used topically. (Araneo) When applied within one hour after injury, DHEA preserved immunocompetency. Their capacity to produce T-cell-derived lymphokines and to generate cellular immune-responses was completely normal. Animal studies for a model for the development of lupus showed that the production of auto-antibodies was significantly restrained by DHEA treatment.

Dr. Jim McGuire, Associate Professor of Medicine at Stanford University of Medicine, is currently conducting a clinical trial of DHEA in patients with lupus.

DHEA is also being tested in patients with multiple sclerosis. Preliminary findings indicate that DHEA produces significant improvement in stamina and a sense of well being in people suffering from multiple sclerosis. (Calabrese, Isaacs, Regelson)

## Rheumatoid Arthritis

Dr. Davis Lamson, a private practitioner in Kent, Washington, has seen exciting results with DHEA in various autoimmune disorders. He finds that serum levels of DHEA are often toward the lower end of normal in people with rheumatoid arthritis or ulcerative colitis. Lamson has given DHEA to six patients with ulcerative colitis who had failed to respond to other types of treatments. In all six cases, the bleeding, diarrhea, and overall condition improved. Lamson has also determined that DHEA therapy is valuable in treating rheumatoid arthritis and other forms of arthritis when the initial DHEA levels are low. (Lamson)

DHEA levels have also been found to be low in women with rheumatoid arthritis, a condition frequently associated with osteoporosis. In a study of forty-nine postmenopausal women with rheumatoid arthritis, DHEA levels (measured as DHEA-S) were significantly lower than in healthy controls. (Sambrotk)

DHEA levels were reduced to a greater extent in women taking corticosteroids (cortisone-like drugs) for their arthritis than in those who were not. That finding is not surprising since administering these drugs is known to reduce the levels of adrenal androgens such as DHEA. (Sambrotk)

However, DHEA levels were also significantly reduced in arthritic women who were not receiving corticosteroids. In this group of forty-nine women, DHEA levels correlated significantly with bone mineral density of the neck of the femur (a bone in the hip) and the spine. The serum level of DHEA was able to predict bone mineral density even after corticosteroid therapy was taken into account. This study suggests that DHEA might be of benefit to people with rheumatoid arthritis.

Supplementing with DHEA might prevent the osteoporosis that so often develops in individuals with rheumatoid arthritis, particularly in those who are taking corticosteroids. In addition, DHEA may impact positively on the arthritic process itself. According to Dr. Iamson, who has given DHEA to several arthritic patients with low serum levels of DHEA, this treatment often relieves pain and morning stiffness, increases strength, and reduces the need for anti-inflammatory medication. In a study of 45 postmenopausal women being treated with corticosteroids, administering DHEA (20 mg/day) resulted in an increased sense of well-being, with no side effects. (Crilly)

# Chronic Fatigue Syndrome

Chronic Fatigue Syndrome, commonly associated with Epstein Barr Virus, and may also be associated with other viruses, has been a medical challenge as conventional treatment has, for the most part, been unsatisfactory. It is a debilitating condition becoming increasingly prevalent among young and middle-aged adults.

Nutrition-oriented doctors have had some success treating Chronic Fatigue Syndrome with allergy diets, thyroid hormones, L-Carnitine, nutrient injections (particularly magnesium and B-vitamins), and other treatments. When DHEA is given to individuals whose energy levels are low-normal or below normal, in a number of cases it has produced definite improvement in energy level, stamina, and general well being.

# DHEA Therapy and AIDS

Epidemiological studies provide evidence that reduced serum levels of DHEA are related to the progression of AIDS in HIV-1 infection. DHEA has also been shown to inhibit HIV-1 replication in vitro and block HIV-1. Abnormally low blood levels of DHEA are associated with increased progression of HIV infection. (Jacobson)

DHEA levels are reduced in people infected with HIV and these levels decline even more as the disease progresses to full-blown AIDS. In a recent study, 108 HIV-positive men with marginally low helper T-cell counts (between 200 and 499) were observed. Men with serum DHEA levels below normal were 2.34 times as likely to progress to AIDS as were those with normal DHEA levels. (Jacobson) These studies provide evidence that a deficiency may be one of the factors contributing to immune system failure. (Merril)

Clinical trials are underway for the use of DHEA as an adjunct HIV therapy. (Henderson)

## DHEA Fights AZT- Resistant HIV

One of the major obstacles to deal with among individuals with acquired immunodeficiency syndrome is HIV-1 resistance to AZT, which occurs after one or two years of treatment. AZT also has significant toxic side effects, further limiting its use in the therapy of HIV-1-infected individuals.

DHEA has demonstrated a broad spectrum of biological functions. It is bioavailable orally and relatively nontoxic. Researchers at the Department of Microbiology and Immunology, Temple University School of Medicine, Philadelphia, PA, investigated whether DHEA treatment could inhibit replication of AZT-resistant strains of HIV-1 Addition of DHEA to MT-2 cell cultures infected with either AZT-sensitive or AZT-resistant isolates of HIV-1 resulted in dose-dependent inhibition of HIV-1-demonstrated suppression of HIV-1 replication.

At a concentration as low as 50 mg, DHEA reduced AZT-resistant HIV-1 replication over 50 percent. This study provides evidence that DHEA can inhibit the replication of AZT-resistant as well as the "wild-type" HIV-1.

Since the main targets for DHEA are metabolic and cellular signaling pathways leading to HIV-1 replication-activation, the researchers stated that DHEA should be effective against multi drug-resistant strains of HIV-1. (Yang, Schwart, Henderson)

In addition, DHEA has shown to enhance the immune response to numerous additional viral infections.

DHEA also has inhibitory effects on Epstein-Barr Virus. It stimulates DNA synthesis in human lymphocytes (protective bacterial and virus-fighting white blood cells). (Henderson) When mice were given a lethal dose of a toxin, mortality was reduced from 95 to 24 percent by treatment with a single dose of DHEA. (Danenberg)

## Chapter Summary

DHEA has a number of varied beneficial effects on the immune system and against a number of degenerative and infectious diseases. DHEA stimulates T-cells, B-cells, and macrophages by interfering with glucocorticoid immuno-suppression. DHEA protects against both bacterial and viral infections. Research in areas such as lupus, multiple sclerosis, chronic fatigue and AIDS shows great promise. In general, most people taking DHEA report feelings of increased tolerance to stress, fatigue and illness.

# DHEA: WEIGHT LOSS, DIABETES & HEART DISEASE

Supplemental DHEA has a wide range of interrelated beneficial effects in the body. This is of additional significance because many degenerative conditions are related in that the existence of one condition can cause an increase risk for development of another. For example, obesity is a risk factor for diabetes. Both obesity and diabetes are risk factors for the development of cardiovascular disease. These three conditions share a common characteristic in that elevated glucose levels are seen. Glucose, a simple sugar molecule derived from carbohydrates, is the primary source of energy in the body. DHEA has a beneficial effect on the manner in which glucose is utilized. DHEA also improves fat metabolism, protects the arteries, and much more. This substance is bound to receive a great deal more attention in these areas in the very near future.

## DHEA Fights Against Obesity

One of the most striking effects of DHEA is its ability to induce weight loss in laboratory animals, even when these animals are given as much food as they want. This remarkable finding by Dr. Arthur Schwartz (Temple University Medical School) in the 1980s produced tremendous interest in the possibility of using DHEA as a weight loss therapy in humans. Recent research has begun to show how DHEA exerts its extraordinary weight loss effects.

## DHEA Speeds Up Metabolism

Animal studies suggest that DHEA may be very effective in treating obesity. In a strain of mice that has a genetic predisposition to obesity, administering DHEA at a dose three times a week of 500 mg per kg (2.2lbs) of dietary consumption, prevented the development of obesity. DHEA did not cause any toxic effects and did not suppress appetite, indicating that its effect was to speed up the metabolism. (Yen)

In another study, administering DHEA (0.6 percent of the diet) decreased body weight and body fat in both lean and obese Zucker rats. The decrease in body fat was primarily due to a decrease in the number of fat cells in lean rats and to decreases in both the number and size of fat cells in obese rats. (Cleary)

"Energy wastage" is thought to be one of the ways that DHEA reduces body weight. In a study with rats, DHEA seemed to exert part of its anti-obesity and anti-diabetic effects through increased liver-glucose oxidation and reduced gluconeogenesis. Gluconeogenesis is the process by which the body converts stored glycogen to glucose so that it can be burned by the body for energy. Excess calories are converted to glycogen in the liver and stored to be burned later when needed. Obesity and diabetes are characterized by high levels of glucose occurring in spite of increased levels of insulin.

Insulin instructs glucose to enter the cells to be burned (oxidized) for energy. In both insulin resistant mutant mice and in normal aging mice, DHEA increases sensitivity to insulin, thereby potentiating its effects of increasing metabolism or glucose burning. (Coleman) In this way, DHEA helps burn those excess calories instead of storing them as glycogen.

DHEA lessens the effects of diabetes in disease prone mice. Rats genetically predisposed to diabetes do not develop the disease when given DHEA, nor do they suffer damage to "islet cells" which produce insulin in the pancreas when given DHEA. (Gordon) Some clinicians report that DHEA treatment reduces the need for insulin in humans.

## DHEA Reduces Desire to Eat

A recent study in diabetes prone rats indicates that one of DHEA's weight reducing mechanisms may operate through the increase of serotonin levels in the hypothalamus region of the brain, thereby increasing the release of cholecystokinin, the satiation hormone. This hormone reduces one's desire for food by creating a feeling of "fullness." DHEA fed rats showed an increase in serotonin levels in the hypothalamus. This was associated with increased activity of this satiation hormone which reduced food intake and lowered body fat.

DHEA's effects on satiation may also be related to its beneficial regulatory effects on insulin and blood sugar. When blood sugar levels drop, a signal is sent to the brain telling you to eat.

## DHEA Prevents Fat Storage

DHEA helps EXPEND energy rather than store it as fat. DHEA inhibits fat synthesis and deposition. (Berdanier) DHEA can prevent obesity in mice genetically predisposed to obesity. When given DHEA the body weights of genetically obese mice reached that of lean mice independent of any alteration in food intake. (Yen) Even middle aged genetically obese mice were thin after given DHEA. (Cleary) Rats whose obesity had been induced by a high-calorie diet, lost weight rapidly when treated with DHEA. DHEA also produced lipid and insulin lowering effects. (Mohan)

## DHEA Works Against Hormone Which Promotes Fat-Storage

DHEA is believed to produce its anti-obesity effects by its anti-glucocorticoid activity. (Wright) Glucocorticoid is a hormone produced by the adrenal glands which aids carbohydrate processing by stimulating the conversion of excess glucose to stored glycogen.

Normally, secretion is brought on by low blood sugar and by the growth hormone. Glucocorticoids aid the release of stored fatty acids and amino acids from muscle. A deficiency is marked by weight loss, low blood sugar, and lack of energy. An excess is linked to damaged sugar digestion, problems with excess weight, and fat storage.

In one study using rats, DHEA blocked the activity of the glucocorticoid-induced enzymes in genetically obese rats leading to substantial weight loss in these animals. Thereby, DHEA, again, seemed to promote burning of the glucose instead of allowing it to be stored. (Riley)

## DHEA Increases Fat Metabolism

DHEA contributes to potential weight loss through a variety of mechanisms. (Cleary, Lardy, Berdainer, McIntosh, MacEwen, Schwartz)

Neuroendocrine control of fat metabolism mediated by DHEA suggests that DHEA circulating levels could serve as a communicating system with the hypothalamus to determine the size of fat stores. (Kurtz) DHEA is freely diffusible into fat stores. The increased response of DHEA to ACTH in simple obesity provides additional evidence.

DHEA can block corticosteroid responses. (Riley) In that regard, CRF stimulates the release of ACTH, cortisol, and DHEA in pubertal development. DHEA acts as a factor in enhanced energy loss and fat mobilization.

High doses of DHEA were given to five normal weight males at a dose of 1,500 mg per day divided into four doses. After 28 days, with diet and physical activity remaining normal, four of the five exhibited a mean body fat decrease of 31 percent with no overall weight change.

This meant that their fat loss was balanced by a gain in muscle mass characteristic of youth! At the same time, the LDL levels fell by 7.5 percent which protects them against cardiovascular disease. (Nester)

A study on DHEA and visceral fat accumulation (fat surrounding the internal organs in the body) in relation to sex hormones in obese men and women undergoing weight loss therapy, showed a correlation among women, but not men. The study included 70 healthy obese men and premenopausal women, aged 27-51, on a diet for 13 weeks.

In women, an abundance of visceral fat was significantly associated with diminished levels of sex hormone-binding globulin and free beta-estradiol/free testosterone ratio and to elevated levels of free testosterone. Loss of visceral fat was significantly related to rises in the sex hormone-binding globulin level and the free 17 beta-estradiol/free testosterone ratio independent of total fat loss. In obese men, sex steroid levels appear not to depend on the amount of visceral fat. (Leenen)

There are also a number of additional effects of DHEA on the body which may induce weight loss and fat reduction, including its effects on thyroid hormone function. *Note:* Individuals using wild yam cream who were also taking thyroid supplements have reported the necessity to decrease their dosage of thyroid hormone.

# DHEA Reverses Diabetes

A certain inbred strain of mice have a genetic disorder that causes them to develop diabetes. Their pancreatic beta cells, those cells in the pancreas that make insulin, are spontaneously destroyed during the course of their lifetime. When this strain of mice was given 0.4 percent DHEA in their diet, the diabetes was rapidly reversed and the beta cells were preserved. In a study of other animals without this genetic disorder, DHEA reduced the severity of diabetes resulting from administering the diabetes-inducing chemical, streptozotocin. (Coleman)

Decreased testosterone and DHEA concentrations are associated with increased insulin and glucose concentrations in nondiabetic men.

Many studies indicate that high amounts of the male "androgenic" hormones are associated with insulin resistance and hyper-insulinemia in both premenopausal and postmenopausal women. Increased testosterone and DHEA levels are associated with the opposite effect in men, lower insulin concentrations.

In men, studies show that the association of sex hormone-binding globulin, testosterone, DHEA, and estradiol levels to levels of glucose and insulin are the following:

1. Low testosterone and low DHEA concentrations significantly indicated low insulin levels.

2. Free testosterone and DHEA are significantly inverse ly correlated with glucose concentrations.

3. After adjustment for age, obesity, and body fat distribution, insulin concentrations remained significantly inversely correlated with free testosterone, total testosterone, and DHEA. (Haffner)

Diabetics suffer a higher incidence of cardiovascular disease than individuals with normal carbohydrate metabolism. Recent studies suggest than one cause of increased cardiovascular disease in diabetics may be reduced levels of DHEA caused by high levels of insulin. DHEA's multiple antiatherogenic effects are therefore non-existent when levels are abnormally low in diabetics. Since aging and obesity are both characterized by hyperinsulinemic insulin resistance, it is quite possible that the dramatically increased incidence of adult-onset diabetes and weight gain in older adults may be caused, in part, by the decline in DHEA levels with advancing age. (Nester)

Enhanced adrenocortical activity is a contributing factor to non-insulin dependent diabetes mellitus in women with elevated levels of adrenalcorticol steroids (cortisol, DHEA, etc.). The high sugar levels of the diabetic patients were not related to their elevated testosterone levels or to their degree of insulin resistance, but were significantly associated with an elevated secretion of the adrenalcortical hormones, which, in turn, were associated with postreceptor defects in insulin action. These findings suggest that enhanced adrenocortical activity may be an important factor underlying the development of diabetes in women. (Buffington)

Many studies have shown a significant association between the magnitude of insulin resistance and the plasma insulin levels in non-diabetic patients. All major cardiovascular risk factors are associated with the presence of hyper-insulinemia or insulin resistance. However, studies have not addressed the possible metabolic differences in insulin action that can occur in patients with and without heart disease. Patients with heart disease have the highest level of fasting insulin compared with other patients and the lowest insulin-mediated stimulation in non-oxidative glucose metabolism.

Fasting lipid oxidation was similar in the three groups, but a stronger insulin-mediated inhibition in the control patients was found. In patients with and without coronary heart disease, but with similar risk factors, a significant reduction in non-oxidative glucose metabolism occurs; nevertheless, such impaired glucose handling seems to be worsened in the presence of heart disease. (Paolisso)

# DHEA's Anti-Atherosclerosis Effects

Heart disease is the number one cause of death in the U.S. Elevated cholesterol levels, poor diet, hypertension, obesity, diabetes, cigarette smoking, a history of stroke and/or thromboembolic disease, family history of premature coronary heart disease, and sedentary lifestyle are among the many contributing factors contributing to the development of atherosclerosis. Women with diabetes and hypertension have a greater risk effect for atherosclerosis compared to men.

DHEA levels are an accurate indicator of arterial blockage, dangerous cholesterol levels, hypertension and other risk factors associated with heart disease, especially in men.

## DHEA Levels Lower Among Those at High Risk for Heart Attack

Acute heart attacks are associated with low levels of DHEA and low levels of high density lipoprotein (HDL), the "good" cholesterol. (Salmeron) DHEA has demonstrated to prevent induced hypertension in rats. (Shafagoj) In a study spanning nearly two decades, men's DHEA levels were found to be lower in patients who died of coronary heart disease compared to the levels of controls. (LaCroix) When DHEA levels were measured in 103 middle-aged males undergoing elective coronary angiography, the lowest levels of DHEA corresponded to the greatest arterial blockage.

In contrast, in 103 women studied, no association was noted between DHEA levels and coronary disease. (Herrington)

| DHEA Level | HDL Cholesterol | LDL Cholesterol | Risk for Heart Attack |
|:---:|:---:|:---:|:---:|

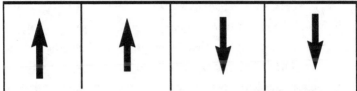

*Lower DHEA levels are associated with lower HDL, high LDL and a higher risk for heart attack.*

| ↑ | ↑ | ↓ | ↓ |
|:---:|:---:|:---:|:---:|

*Higher DHEA levels are associated with higher HDL, low LDL and a lower risk for heart attack.*

In yet another study of 32 men, aged 26-40 years, low levels of DHEA were found in men who had suffered myocardial infarction at least three to four months prior to the study. (Slowinska, Srzednicka)

A study published years ago in *The New England Journal of Medicine* showed that DHEA may play a role in preventing heart disease. Plasma levels of DHEA-S were measured in 242 men, ages 50 to 79. (DHEA-S is easier to measure and provides a rough estimate of DHEA levels.)

In 1986 Elizabeth Barrett-Connor, an epidemiologist at the University of California, San Diego, reported that among 143 middle-aged and elderly men who had been followed for twelve years, the ones with high DHEA-S levels suffered half as many cases of heart disease as the men with low DHEA-S levels. Among men with healthy hearts, those who had low levels of DHEA were 3.3 times more likely to die of heart disease during the next twelve years than those with normal DHEA levels. Women in the study who had high DHEA sulfate levels had a slight higher risk of heart disease. (Barrett-Connor)

Administering DHEA has shown to lower serum LDL-cholesterol, the "bad" form of cholesterol, which is associated with heart disease. These results raise the possibility that in individuals with low DHEA levels, supplementing with DHEA may help prevent heart disease.

## DHEA Discourages Plaque Formation

In a study at Johns Hopkins Medical Institute, DHEA administration retarded arterial plaque formation by almost 50 percent and significantly retarded the progression of atherosclerosis!

DHEA was incorporated into the diet of one group of hyper-cholesterolemic rabbits receiving the 2 percent cholesterol diet with damaged arteries to encourage the formation of atherosclerotic plaque. After 12 weeks the aortas, hearts, and livers were studied and compared to controls. Severe atherosclerosis was seen in animals not treated with DHEA. In those receiving DHEA there was an almost 50 percent reduction in plaque size inversely related to the serum level of DHEA attained. Fatty infiltration of the heart and liver were also markedly reduced. The results show that high levels of plasma DHEA inhibit the development of atherosclerosis, and they provide an important experimental link to epidemiologic studies correlating low DHEA-S plasma levels with an enhanced risk of cardiovascular mortality. (Gordon)

This finding is especially important to those who have undergone coronary-bypass surgery because grafted blood vessels are especially susceptible to new plaque formation. These studies have been reinforced by the epidemiologic work of Barret-Connor, Cleary, MacEwen, Arad, Sonka, Lopez and Nestler.

DHEA has also demonstrated to protect the aortic graft by delaying the arteriosclerotic vascular injury to prevent host graft rejection. If these clinical effects seen are physiologic, replacement therapy to reproduce youthful blood levels would be in order.

# DHEA Lowers LDL and Total Cholesterol

A number of studies show the effect of DHEA on cholesterol biosynthesis. (Schulz) Supplemental oral DHEA-S intake can lower total serum cholesterol, particularly LDL (low density lipoprotein) cholesterol, by an average of 18 percent. The decrease in total cholesterol without changing food intake, activity level, or body weight occurs. (Haffa)

Clinical observations suggests that DHEA may control the phospholipid content of cell membranes. As LDL is the major DHEA serum transporter, DHEA might control cholesterol transport or cell membrane fluidity through LDL. Or, DHEA may affect phospholipid cholesterol ratios in the cell matrix or on the endothelial surface. (Sholley)

In regard to the effects of fat mobilization induced by DHEA as a factor in the prevention of atherosclerosis, an inverse correlation has been found between low-density lipoprotein cholesterol and DHEA. In this regard, researchers have reported a decrease in DHEA levels associated with elevated cholesterol levels. (Biozel)

# DHEA Blocks Enzyme and Oxidation Associated with LDL Cholesterol

DHEA blocks the activity of a rate controlling enzyme, glucose-6-pd dehydrogenase (G6PDH), needed for cellular proliferation and O2 formation. O2 oxidation of LDL cholesterol can create free radicals which are very damaging to the arterial wall. Damaged areas of the arterial walls provide ideal places for plaque to build up. DHEA blockage of this enzyme helps inhibit rapid multiplication of smooth muscle cells such as at the injury site of the arterial wall. (Schwartz)

# DHEA Protects Tissue from Damage

When a person suffers a heart attack (called ischemia-restriction of blood flow to the coronary arteries), the heart muscle is at risk of damage from the return of blood to the affected region (called reperfusion). According to the results of a recent study, DHEA may help protect against such injury. Rats were given DHEA and then subjected to ischemia-reperfusion. In the control rats not receiving DHEA, the muscle tissue with blood flow restriction showed a 69 percent reduction in functional capillary density. Total cessation (0 percent reflow) occurred within 24 hours.

Animals pretreated with DHEA had a temporary 39 percent reduction in functional capillary density. Yet all muscle tissue remained viable when 100 percent reflow resumed. DHEA pretreatment improved microcirculation and protected muscle tissue against damage. (Lohman, R.)

# DHEA Has Different Effects in Men and Women

DHEA has either estrogen-like or androgen-like effects depending on the hormonal environment it is introduced into. DHEA is either an estrogen antagonist, estradiol to estrogen receptor, or an androgen through its metabolism to androstenedione (which converts to the estrogen and testosterone sex hormones) and testosterone.

In premenopausal women with high estrogen levels, DHEA contributes to abdominal obesity and insulin resistance.

**In postmenopausal women with low estrogen levels:** DHEA metabolism to testosterone may increase the risk of cardiovascular disease, though this effect may be counter-balanced by the age-dependent decline in DHEA and also by other estrogen-like effects.

In some breast cancer cell lines, in a low estrogen environment, DHEA has an estradiol-like effect, stimulating tumor growth, whereas where there are high levels of estradiol, DHEA reduces the tumor growth-stimulating effect of estradiol.

**In men:** DHEA, like an estrogen, protects against cardiovascular disease. (Ebeling)

Adrenal androgens and testosterone were investigated as coronary risk factors in the 5-year Helsinki Heart Study. Serum concentrations of DHEA, androstenedione (which converts to the estrogen and testosterone sex hormones), androstanediol glucuronide, cortisol, and testosterones were determined. The findings revealed that DHEA levels were negatively associated with age and HDL-cholesterol.

The association between DHEA and the risk for the development of coronary heart disease was studied using the classical risk factors: age, smoking, blood pressure, and lipid levels. Studies of the joint effects of age and DHEA disclosed that the risk associated with elevated DHEA was confined to older men. A similar analysis with smoking revealed that the DHEA-related risk was mainly found in smokers. A mild steroid biosynthetic defect of the adrenals associated with high DHEA levels increased the coronary heart disease risk in this study population. (Hautanen)

# Heart Disease: Result of Imbalance

Heart disease is a striking example of how our bodies reflect the imbalance of our lifestyle. In the United States, heart disease is the cause of more deaths than all other diseases combined. The incidence of heart attacks has doubled in this country every two decades since 1900 when heart disease was extremely rare. Dr. Paul Dudley White, an eminent cardiologist, believed that the epidemic was due primarily to two changes that had taken

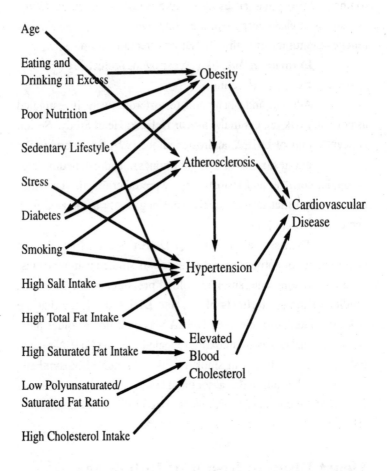

place in America during this century - the enormous "acceleration in the pace of everyday life" and "general enrichment of the diet."

    The automobile greatly decreased the time in which people reached their destinations allowing for pace acceleration, thus came the expression, "the disease of being in a hurry." Instead of walking or biking, we drive cars. Cardiovascular fitness has also become much more difficult in our leisure society, where radio, television and movies have become more popular than exercise.

"Enrichment" basically refers to the diet which contains more fat. After 1920, foods such as butter, cream, and red meat became available not just to the wealthy, but to everyone. This created a particularly unbalanced diet.

If you look around the world, you will see that certain countries have a low incidence of nearly every disease (Japan, Taiwan, Thailand, Salvador) while the United States, Canada, Australia, and Germany have the highest incidence. If you look at the consumption of milk, red meat, eggs, and cheese in these countries, the very same distribution will occur. The nations with low disease rates are those where there is very little consumption of high-fat foods, while those with the rich diets have catastrophic rates of heart disease and cancer, diseases believed by many to be largely preventable.

Hormonal imbalances are also thought to be largely due to a high fat diet, especially the intake of cholesterol. Cholesterol is what hormones are made from in the body. Cholesterol, which we consume when we eat meat, eggs, and dairy products, is produced by the liver. Our liver is able to produce all the body needs and there really is no physiological need for us to obtain any cholesterol at all through the diet.

Some scientists theorize that a high fat diet can trigger over production of some hormones such as estrogen, creating an imbalance. Many women suffer from estrogen dominance, which is characterized by symptoms associated with premenstrual syndrome (PMS), water retention, edema, breast swelling, fibrocystic breasts, premenstrual mood swings, depression, loss of libido, heavy or irregular menses, uterine fibroid, craving for sweets, weight gain, fat deposition at hips and thighs.

While estrogen is believed to have beneficial cardiovascular effects, another synthetic hormone, progestin, exerts a detrimental effect on blood lipids by increasing LDL and reducing HDL cholesterol. Without progestin, prolonged estrogen therapy increases the risk of endometrial cancer. As stated earlier, a balance of all circulating hormones is the key to good health and longevity.

## *Chapter Summary*

DHEA has shown exciting therapeutic effects against obesity in that it encourages weight loss by raising metabolism, decreasing appetite, and discouraging fat storage.

Because of the close relationship between steriod hormone levels and activity of the pancreas, DHEA has shown to reverse diabetes and aid in glucose regulation.

DHEA prevents heart disease because it lowers cholesterol and blocks enzyme activity associated with low density lipoprotein (LDL) oxidation which is associated with plaque formation in the arteries.

# DHEA AGAINST CANCER

Cancer is the abnormal growth of cells in our bodies sufficient to kill us if left untreated. All cancer originates as a change of a normal cell through its genetic chromosome material, RNA and DNA. The cell increases its rate of multiplication. Normally, most cells replicate themselves continually at a rate synchronous with normal growth and repair. Each cell (with the exception of ova and sperm) contains a full complement of chromosomes; yet each develops in a manner specific for its purpose in the body. When a cell becomes cancerous, it multiplies faster than it should and loses normal differentiation.

The actual mechanisms by which cancer is caused is still speculative. It may be the result of DNA damage induced by various stressors such as radiation, viruses or toxins. The body combats this by various repair mechanisms, but, as life progresses, the accumulated bits of damage increase over time weakening our defenses. Thus, the incidence of cancer increases with age. Factors that interfere or impede repair mechanisms predispose one to cancer.

Alcohol
Nitrates
Tobacco, including second-hand smoke
Carbon monoxide
Pesticide residues in food and water
Many pharmaceuticals
Free radicals

Another theory holds that a toxic environment within the cell can stimulate a latent ability of otherwise undamaged chromosomes to change into a more primitive mode of survival in response to threat. This theory suggests that maintaining a healthy intracellular environment will prevent cancer, and that correcting a toxic environment may lead to successful non-toxic treatment for cancer. If this is true, with exposure to known carcinogens, cancer can be prevented by agents such as beta carotene or vitamin C, etc. Numerous studies support this theory.

# Cancer Causing Agents

| _Agents_ | _Estimated Percentage of All Cancers_ |
|---|---|
| Tobacco | 30 percent |
| Natural constituents of food (alfatoxins in peanuts, etc) | 28 percent |
| Sun exposure | 15 percent |
| Sexual and reproductive history | 7 percent |
| Occupational hazards | 4 percent |
| Alcohol | 4 percent |
| Contaminants in air, food and water (Carbon monoxide, radon, formaldehyde, trihalomethanes from chlorine in drinking water, motor vehicle exhaust, chlorofluorcarbons - in refrigerators and conditioners - depleting ozone, etc.) | 4 percent |
| Electrical pollution | 1 percent |
| Unknown | 4 percent |

# Cancer Associated with Low DHEA Levels

Studies indicate an association between DHEA levels and human breast cancer. In one study, urinary excretion of DHEA was below normal in a group of premenopausal women with breast cancer. Other researchers confirmed that DHEA levels are low in premenopausal breast cancer patients, but found that some postmenopausal women with breast cancer had elevated DHEA levels. It appeared that the low levels in the premenopausal patients were due primarily to decreased production while the elevated levels in the postmenopausal patients were due to delayed breakdown. Whatever the reason for the changes, these studies suggest a possible role for DHEA in the prevention or treatment of at least some cases of breast cancer.

Studies indicate that the risk of developing a wide variety of cancers is directly related to the blood or urinary levels of DHEA. In laboratory studies DHEA has prevented the occurrence of many different types of spontaneous and chemically induced tumors including:

> **Colon** (Schultz)
>
> **Lung** (Pashko)
>
> **Skin** (Pashko)
>
> **Breast** (Viral-induced-Schwartz)
>
> (Radiation-induced-Inano)
>
> **Lymphatic** (Risdon)

**Types of cancers associated with low levels of DHEA:**

Gastric cancer (Gordon)

Prostate cancer (Stahl)

Bladder cancer (Gordon)

Breast cancer (Bulbrook)

Ovarian cancer

# DHEA Prevents Cancer

DHEA shows great promise as an anticancer agent. DHEA has shown to inhibit the development of tumors and other disorders of rodents. In mice that develop spontaneous breast cancer, long-term administration of DHEA prevented the cancer from occurring. Treatment of mice with DHEA delayed the appearance of colon tumors resulting from administering a carcinogen. (Nyce) DHEA inhibited the development of liver cancer in rats treated with chemical carcinogens. (Mayer)

One of the most interesting aspects of supplemental DHEA is its ability to suppress "overactive" body processes. These include over-production of nucleic acids, fats, hormones, and cells which may be considered cancerous.

### *Examples of cancer protective means through DHEA:*

**1.** Enhances immune activity

**2.** Inhibits fat formation.

**3.** Slows free radical formation by blocking 02 formation.

**4.** Slows proliferation of pre-cancerous tissue/Prevents tumor cell proliferation

**5.** Reduces synthesis of mutagenic cells.

**6.** Converts to androgens. (Risdon)

DHEA supplementation is also associated with a reduction in glucose consumption (reduces sugar cravings), and increases the use of stored glycogen (prevents fat from getting stored and burns stored energy).

DHEA increases the efficiency of DNA repair to the effects of radiation used as a cancer treatment of mutagenesis. Depending on the timing of DHEA administration to whole body radiation, DHEA has radiation protective and/or enhancing

action. Similar protection is seen for DHEA in stimulating mutagenic repair mechanisms.

# DHEA Blocks Cell Rate Controlling Enzyme

Much of the anticarcinogenic effects of supplemental
DHEA is due to its effects on cellular growth and mutagenesis.
DHEA blocks glucose-6-pd dehydrogenase (G6PDH). This is a
rate-controlling enzyme needed for cellular carcinogen activation,
cellular proliferation, and O2 formation. High G6PDH enzyme
activity is seen in precancerous and cancerous cells of the colon,
skin, mouth, liver, etc. Blockage of this enzyme inhibits carcinogen synthesis and prevents a cellular invader from doing any
damage or going any further. (VanNoorden) This enzyme is necessary for growth of the tumor, and if we could stop its activities,
we could stop the tumor growth. (Feo, Pascale) This is exactly
what DHEA does. DHEA inhibits G6PDH enzyme activity. (Feo/
Pascale, Schwartz/Pashiko)

### DHEA: The Ultimate Antioxidant

DHEA can block cancer during its early sates as though
its blocking action of G6PDH, it also disarms NADPH, an
enzyme that activates carcinogens and generates oxygen free radicals. Oxygen free radicals may contribute to many other age-
related diseases besides cancer, such as atherosclerosis and neuro-
degenerative disorders. The antioxidant actions of DHEA offer a
multitude of benefits. (Schwartz, Jesse and Whitcomb)

# DHEA and Dietary Restriction

The protective effects of DHEA are tin some ways
thought to be similar to the effects of dietary restriction which
increases intracellular immunity against carcinogens. (Schwartz)

Long-term DHEA treatment of mice also reduces

weight gain (apparently by enhancing thermogenesis) and appears to produce many of the beneficial effects of food restriction which have been shown to inhibit the development of many age-associated diseases including cancer. (Schwartz)

Recent work in the anti-aging, life-extending mechanism of dietary restriction in rodents is thought to be due to the lowering of body temperature during sleep. The evidence suggests that this temperature fall enhances the ability of DNA to repair itself which decreases abnormalities.

Many years ago it was discovered that reducing the food intake of mice increases the activity of the adrenal cortex. One might speculate that elevated levels of DHEA could possibly be contributing to the age-retarding effects of food restriction. (Boutwell)

In further support of DHEA anticarcinogenesis effect paralleling dietary restriction, especially created synthetic DHEA derivatives which do not have sex steroid action are three times more potent as anti-obesity agents than regular DHEA. (Hastings)

# Hormonally-Responsive Tumors

Research has not yet fully determined the relationship between DHEA and hormonally-responsive tumors. It is recognized that DHEA is a sensitive indicator that can distinguish presence of cancerous tissues.

### DHEA: Caution Regarding Prostate

Because of the similarity to other sex hormones, there is some concern that DHEA might cause prostate enlargement, but not all scientists are in agreement on this. (Regelson) Most clinicians caution, however, that DHEA therapy should not be used when there are prostate abnormalities, because some DHEA is converted to testosterone, which could potentially worsen this condition. Some researchers suggest that inhibitors such as Proscar or Permixon, which block the conversion of testosterone to dihydro-testosterone, could lessen this detrimental effect on the prostate gland.

## Cancerous Breast Tissue Contains Less DHEA

The levels of DHEA-S found in normal breast fluid in women exceeds blood plasma levels by 50 to 1,000 times. For this reason, there has been some concern that its conversion to estrogen might promote tumor growth. Animal studies have shown that DHEA can both block and stimulate mammary tumor growth. It has also been suggested that DHEA may act as both a promoter and a suppressor of breast tumors for pre- and post-menopausal women. More studies must be done to clarify this. (Regelson)

Sex steroids have a long history in suppressing the growth of breast tumors. Supplemental DHEA can slow some types of human breast cancer cell growth where it affects the availability of enzymes necessary for tumor proliferation.

Of interest to clinical cancer therapy is that these steroids, along with their proliferative effect, induce progesterone specific binding sites in these estrogen sensitive cell lines suggesting that following DHEA priming, progesterone or progesterone antagonists could influence breast tumor growth.

## DHEA Reduces Breast Cancer

Supplemental DHEA significantly decreased mammary tumors in laboratory animals by 35 percent. The first appearance of tumors in the DHEA-fed group was 4.5 months later than in the control group. Hormone levels in the serum of DHEA-fed rats showed estrogen levels 6 times higher than the control rats without supplemental DHEA, while the levels of progesterone and prolactin were decreased by 30 and 45 percent, respectively.

Interestingly, DHEA prevented hypertrophy of the pituitary, but stimulated the development of mammary glands more than that in control rats. These findings suggest that DHEA has a potent preventive activity against the promotion/progression phase of radiation-induced mammary tumorigenesis. (Inano)

In other studies, DHEA has also shown considerable therapeutic potential for the treatment of breast cancer. Evidence suggests that the DHEA-S may have a crucial role in regulating cytokine production and that this may indirectly control tumor estrogen synthesis. (Reed)

## *Some interesting findings:*

● Breast cancer patients who have below normal blood levels and urinary excretion levels of DHEA indicate poor prognosis. (Bulbrook) Breast cancer patients with high DHEA/cortisol plasma ratios respond well to endocrine therapy. Some researchers feel that this information can be used to predict response of an individual to treatment. (O'Higgins)

● Some researchers have reported that DHEA has an antagonistic effect to stress-mediated corticosteroid action which can affect tumor growth or immuno-response related to tumor/host resistance.

● Breast cancer tissue in-vitro can convert DHEA to hydroxy-DHEA and androstenediol (AED). It is thought that AED can compete with estrogen for estrogen receptors which may provoke proliferative action and that DHEA conversion to AED may play a role in the "western high fat" pattern of breast cancer.

● DHEA anti-tumor relationships is a function of G-6-PD enzyme inhibition. This is supported by the fact that in individuals where G-6-PD deficiencies are a genetic problem, there is a decreased incidence of cancer. (Feo and Pascale)

● A correlation exists between DHEA and potassium concentration in breast cysts. A decrease in DHEA in high sodium cyst fluid may relate to antibody cross reacting steroids.

● In individuals with ovarian tumors the circulating levels of DHEA are clinically lower than normal. However, one study described an ovarian tumor which produced large concentrations of DHEA. (Barkan) Paradoxically, in another study, DHEA induced ovarian tumors in the research mice. In this model, the DHEA systemic effect on vaginal epithelium was estrogenic and testosterone enhanced tumor incidence, but estradiol inhibited it.

● DHEA has also shown to protect the kidneys from carcinogenesis against nitrosamines, while it is not protective against lung cancer with the same carcinogen. (Moore)

## Topical DHEA Inhibits Skin Cancer

Skin cancer is the most common form of cancer today. If detected early, it usually can be treated, however, it can be deadly. The New York Academy of Sciences recently reported a study done years ago by Drs. Arthur Schwartz and Laura Pashko. They found that in addition to DHEA's inhibition of a number of other types of cancer, topical application of DHEA on mouse skin inhibited the promotion of skin papillomas and melanoma. While the papillomas were chemically induced, the study none-the-less demonstrated great potential for an additional therapeutic application for DHEA. More studies need to be done in this exciting area. (Schwartz, Pashko "Cancer Prevention and DHEA" New York Academy of Sciences (1996) pages 180-186.)

## DHEA and Radiation

DHEA seems to have a protective effect on the body against radiation. DHEA given to mice 0-16 hours before radiation showed a protective effect at 30 days. In contrast, if DHEA was given 20-52 hours before radiation, individuals were more sensitive to radiation. This study was based upon the observation that liver glucose-6-PD enzyme was inhibited in mice subjected to sub-lethal whole body irradiation which had effects which were felt could be critical to radiation repair. (Sonka and Strakova)

Of interest to the above, both DHEA and progesterone have protective effects on genetic chromosomal materials following exposure to mutagens in mice. This again suggests that DHEA may stimulate anti-mutagenic or DNA repair mechanisms in the body. (Wilpart)

## Chapter Summary

DHEA protects against a number of various types of cancers including colon, lung, skin, breast, and lymphatic. Protection from these cancers was obtained because DHEA inhibits fat formation, slows free radical formation, slows proliferation of pre-cancerous tissue, reduces synthesis of mutagenic cells or possibly relates to the fact that DHEA converts to androgens. Caution is advised for individuals who are under high risk for hormonally responsive tumors such as prostate cancer. More information is needed to determine their relationship with DHEA.

# DHEA AND THE BRAIN

Much of the excitement about DHEA and longevity is that it makes people <u>feel better</u>. Testimonials from individuals using DHEA range from statements like:

*"I slept less, but I felt better."*

*"I just feel more able to cope with life's stresses and challenges."*

*"The change in my libido was so striking that both my wife and I noticed. I feel like I am twenty years old again." (Note: This man, taking DHEA for 6 years, is 70 years old. He doesn't look a day over 50, and could probably pass for 45.)*

*"I felt more energy. I just jumped out of bed in the morning."*

*"It seemed to give me more energy, more glow."*

*"I simply felt younger, more alive."*

It's much easier to grow old gracefully when you feel better, feel younger, and feel healthier. It's hard to do anything if you feel tired and depressed. These mental effects of DHEA may indeed reflect the physiological effects that DHEA has on the body. But DHEA definitely has direct effects on the brain itself.

DHEA is found in high levels in the brain in concentrations equal to that in the adrenal cortex. Cerebral spinal fluid contains about 5 percent of what is found in the blood. The brain depends on neurotransmitter chemicals which allow communication between brain cells (neurons). Low levels of DHEA are an indication of lower levels of neurons.

With age, fewer neurotransmitters are produced and the ability to "communicate" is reduced. Neurotransmitters (such as acetylcholine, norepinephrine and serotonin) affect sexual desire, emotions, memory and learning. Low levels of any of these can cause forgetfulness, inability to concentrate, sleeplessness and sleep disorders, (such as the inability to fall or stay asleep, which is common in older persons), depression, and muscle incoordination.

Diet can also affect production of neurotransmitters. For production, the brain requires the B-complex vitamins, choline and pantothenic acid, as well as the amino acids, tryptophan, phenylalanine and tyrosine.

## Dementia and Alzheimer's Disease

Alzheimer's patients have lower levels of DHEA than individuals of the same age group who do not have Alzheimer's. Recently it was reported that levels of DHEA were on average 48 percent lower in individuals with Alzheimer's Disease compared to age-matched controls, which in turn, were approximately 50 percent lower than those of younger controls. (Sunderland) Studies have also shown that DHEA levels are exceedingly low at ages when the incidence of Alzheimer's Disease begins to increase markedly.

Supplemental DHEA is believed to relieve memory loss that contributes to dementia or is caused by it. (Nasman)

The role that DHEA plays in Alzheimer's and memory restoration is not yet fully determined. DHEA may play a significant role in maintaining the function of neuronal cells, and DHEA supplementation may prevent neuronal loss and/or damage, thus showing the progress of Alzheimer's disease. (Bologa)

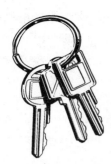

## Can DHEA help you find your keys?

# Maybe!

An age related decline in circulating brain levels of DHEA can be correlated with declining levels of potassium channel functions.

## Cognition, Memory, and Learning

DHEA appears to have the ability to restore memory by encouraging brain cell formation.

A study with men residing in nursing homes, ages 57-104, compared to men of similar ages living independently outside the nursing home, showed a significant and interesting relationship in DHEA levels to degree of dependence. The study reported that plasma DHEA levels were inversely related to the presence of organic brain syndrome and to the degree of dependence in performing the activities of daily living. The nursing home men had DHEA levels that were significantly lower than men of similar ages living outside the nursing home. There were 40 percent subnormal DHEA levels in the nursing home men compared to only 6 percent subnormal DHEA levels for the outside men. Plasma DHEA was subnormal in 80 percent of the nursing home men who had deteriorated to the point where they required total care. (Rudman)

Even small amounts of DHEA were found to lessen amnesia and enhance long-term memory in mice. In vitro studies have shown that small concentrations of supplemental DHEA can enhance brain cells of a mouse. Therefore, the conclusion may be that DHEA compounds might help in the treatment of neuro-degenerative memory disorders in man. (Roberts)

Memory enhancement was achieved by the addition of DHEA to the water supply of mice. Benefits depended on the correct level of DHEA obtained. When too little DHEA was given memory benefits dropped off steeply, as was the case when too much DHEA was given.

Improved memory was found in mice in one study even when DHEA was administered after the learning experience had occurred. DHEA improved memory retention in middle-aged and old mice to the high levels observed in young mice. (Flood)

Even very low levels of DHEA supplementation can increase the number of neurons in the brain, as well as their ability to establish contact with other neurons, and to differentiate. Supplementation with DHEA has also shown to prevent neuronal loss and/or damage. (Bologa)

## Pregnenolone and Memory

Pregnenolone, the precursor to DHEA, has demonstrated its beneficial influence on brain chemistry in numerous ways. Pregnenolone has been found to inhibit the GABA receptors in brain cells, which may result in increased mental alertness. It may also stimulate the NMDA (N-methyl-D-aspartate) receptors, which play an important role in regulating synapses, thus influencing learning and memory.

In 1992, a ground-breaking study was conducted on experimental mice and the supplemental effects of the steroid hormones on memory. Mice were placed in a T-shaped maze and given 5 seconds after a bell sounded to find their way into the correct arm of the T. If they failed to do so within 5 seconds, they were given a mild electric shock until they succeeded. Once trained in the "foot-shock active-avoidance" procedure the mice were injected with a steroid hormone or a placebo. One week later, they were retested for retention of the learned response.

Almost all steroids were found to reduce the number of runs required for the mice to relearn the shock/avoidance procedure (to successfully run the T-maze 5 out of 6 consecutive attempts). Pregnenolone was unique in being active in doses one hundred times lower than any other steroid compound.

Most hormones were found to exhibit an inverted-U-shaped dose response curve which covered a two- to five-fold dose range. DHEA, however, was effective at decreasing the number of runs at doses over a hundred-fold range, and pregnenolone at an up-to-ten-thousand-fold dose range. The scientists were unable to identify the exact mode of the memory-enhancing activity and the structural feature of the different steroids. (Morely)

In another study with mice, it was found that the memory-enhancing effects of DHEA occurred even when DHEA was given one hour after training! In this study, there was improved memory retention over a much wider dose range than is usual for excitatory memory enhancers, giving rise to the idea that DHEA may modulate the transcription of intermediate early genes needed for changes that occur during memory processing.

The memory-enhancing effects of DHEA and pregnenolone in mice have been documented. Infusion of pregnenolone into the rat after the acquisition trial enhanced memory performance in a two-trial recognition task showing a positive correlation between performance and the concentrations of pregnenolone. The animals which performed best had the highest pregnenolone and DHEA levels. (Robel)

## DHEA Decreases Aggressive Behavior

DHEA also inhibited the aggressive behavior of female mice towards lactating female intruders. The degree of inhibition of aggressive behavior was related to the level of decrease of pregnenolone concentrations in brain. (Robel)

# DHEA Lifts Depression

Low thyroid function and depression are closely tied, but whether the low thyroid function is a result of depression or the depression a result of low thyroid function remains to be definitively determined. It is probably a combination. Depressive illness is often a first or early manifestation of thyroid disease, as even subtle decreases in available thyroid hormone are suspected of producing symptoms of depression. Depressed patients should be screened for hypothyroidism, particularly if they complain of fatigue as well.

Like the thyroid gland, dysfunction of the adrenal glands is closely associated with depression. Defects in adrenal function observed in depressed subjects include excessive cortisol secretion, abnormal nocturnal release of cortisol, and inadequate suppression of the secretion of cortisone by the drug dexamethasone.

The psychological effects of increased adrenal release of cortisol mirror the effects of orally administered corticosteroid drugs: depression, mania, nervousness, insomnia, and schizophrenia. The effects of corticosteroids on mood are related to their prevention of serotonin synthesis from tryptophan in the brain.

Subjects suffering from depression were given various forms of pharmacotherapy and behavioral therapy. The DHEA levels of 47 individuals showed a positive correlation with rating scale improvement as their depression was relieved. (Tollefson)

## *Chapter Summary*

People taking DHEA simply claim that they feel better; less stressed, less depressed, more energetic. DHEA has shown to improve memory by increasing formation of brain cells. DHEA has also shown to decrease aggressive behavior and decrease depression. Alzheimer's patients have lower levels of DHEA than individuals of the same age group who do not have Alzheimer's.

# DHEA AND OSTEOPOROSIS

The bone thinning disease, osteoporosis, is responsible for 1.3 million fractures in men and women over age 45. In women, after menopause, osteoporosis becomes more of a problem.

The known factors affecting calcium acquisition and normal bone building are multiple and include the following:. Normal calcium absorption, sufficient gastric acidity and adequate vitamin D. Many older women are deficient in vitamin D due to insufficient sun exposure and many over age 70 lack sufficient gastric acidity.

The incorporation of calcium into normal bone requires bone stress (exercise) and appropriate hormonal control - parathyroid hormone and progesterone. It is important to rule out excess thyroid hormone (not uncommon in women taking thyroid medication) and hypercortisolism, especially in patients given corticosteroids.

The concentration of calcium in the blood is strictly maintained within very narrow limits. If levels start to decrease there is an increase in the secretion of parathyroid hormone and a decrease in the secretion of calcitonin by the thyroid. If calcium levels in the blood start to increase there is a decrease in the secretion of parathyroid hormone and an increase in the secretion of calcitonin. An understanding of how these hormones increase and decrease calcium levels in the blood is necessary in understanding osteoporosis.

Calcitonin decreases calcium levels in the blood.

Parathyroid hormone increases calcium levels primarily by increasing the activity of the cells that break down bone (osteoclasts). It also decreases the excretion of calcium by the kidneys and increases the absorption of calcium in the intestines.

Since bone mass and serum DHEA both decline with advancing age, one cannot be certain that falling DHEA levels are actually the cause of reduced bone mass. However, there is evidence that aging alone cannot explain the relationship between DHEA levels and bone mass. In a recent study of Belgian women, significant correlations were found between bone mineral content and DHEA levels (measured as DHEA-S) even after correcting for the effects of age. (Rozenburg)

In another study serum DHEA levels were significantly lower in 49 women with osteoporosis than in women of similar age without osteoporosis. DHEA levels declined with age in both groups of women. Those with osteoporosis had lower levels of DHEA at all ages. (Nordin) These studies support the proposed role of DHEA in maintaining bone mass.

## Estrogen and Bone Loss

Estrogen deficiency causes bone loss. Osteoclasts (cells that break down bone) become more sensitive to parathyroid hormone, resulting in increased bone breakdown, thereby raising calcium levels in the blood. This leads to a decreased parathyroid hormone level which results in diminished levels of active vitamin D and increased calcium excretion as well.

Calcitonin lowers calcium levels in the blood by simulating osteoblasts (cells that build bone). Low calcitonin levels are found in postmenopausal osteoporosis and are responsible for the bone loss seen among these women. Calcitonin (isolated from salmon) has demonstrated remarkable effects in clinical studies and holds much promise in treating severe osteoporosis. (This is available only by prescription.)

Estrogen stimulates the liver to produce a protein that binds certain adrenal hormones, and lessens their ability to dissolve bone. Low levels of estrogens, which are common after menopause, often contribute to bone loss in women.

However, there is very little osteoporosis among the Bantu women of Africa, even after menopause, which occurs at the same age as American women. Studies show that postmenopausal Bantu women have more estrogen that postmenopausal American women. Why? American women have seemingly upset their body chemistry through diet and other means. Consequently, with age, the hormones do not function as well.

Bantu women consume a minimum of milk, no calcium supplements, and no estrogen pills after menopause. Also, they take in little sugar, caffeine, alcohol, aspirin, corticosteroids, antibiotics, or other drugs. The body stays in homeostasis much of the time and is not continually pulling calcium out of the bones over a lifetime. It is not known if postmenopausal Bantu women experience better thyroid function and other endocrine gland functions compared to American women. Just something to think about...

# Amenorrhea and Bone Density

Amenorrhea (experience of no monthly menstruation) indicates the presence of estrogen deficiency unless a woman is pregnant or has had a hysterectomy. Estrogen deficiency and amenorrhea have many causes: prolactin-producing tumors, anorexia nervosa, intense exercise associated with leanness, as well as natural or surgical menopause. All of these causes for amenorrhea are cross-sectionally associated with low bone density. A low bone density in women with amenorrhea, however, does not indicate whether the cause is an abnormally low peak bone mass or a subsequently accelerated rate of bone loss. There are no prospective data documenting the level of peak bone mass achieved in a cohort of women with primary or secondary amenorrhea compared with women who had normal menstrual maturation.

The data on the rates of bone change in women with amenorrhea is scarce. Cortical bone change rates vary formation and complements estrogen.

## Estrogen Supplementation

Conventional medicine has shown that synthetic estrogen, if used continuously, can temporarily stop further bone loss in osteoporosis victims. But, continuous use of synthetic estrogen increases the risk for cancer, diabetes, high blood pressure, abnormal clotting, AND does nothing to replace lost bone cells. It is generally agreed that the risks outweigh the benefits in the majority of women who are at risk for osteoporosis.

Corticosteroids are known to be an important cause of osteoporosis, perhaps in part, because they deplete DHEA. Would simultaneous administration of DHEA inhibit some of the side effects of corticosteroids, including osteoporosis? Our natural adrenal secretions contain both of these hormones, and nature usually does things for a reason. Animal studies suggest that DHEA does, in fact, modulate some of the negative effects of corticosteroids.

## DHEA Increases Bone Mineral Density

DHEA, like estrogen, progesterone, and testosterone, has been shown to improve osteoporosis. (Mayer) DHEA not only has a direct effect on both resorption and formation of bone, but it can also increase the levels of other major hormones - estrogen, progesterone, and testosterone, important for bone mineral density. Men who have low levels of testosterone have a higher incidence of osteoporosis.

In a study of postmenopausal women, administering DHEA increased serum levels of both testosterone and estrogens. (Regelson)

Although DHEA is not converted directly into progesterone, it may, however, convert through a feedback mechanism. *(See page 30)* Both DHEA and progesterone are produced from the same precursor hormone, pregnenolone. If enough DHEA is present, then pregnenolone will be converted primarily to progesterone, rather than to DHEA.

Administration of DHEA to ovariectomized rats significantly increased bone mineral density. These findings strongly suggest that serum adrenal androgen may be converted to estrogen, and be important steroids to maintain bone mineral density, especially in the sixth to seventh decades after menopause. (Nawata)

## DHEA prevents bone loss in a number of ways:

1. DHEA improves calcium absorption, possibly due to effects on vitamin D metabolism.

2. A breakdown product of DHEA binds to estrogen receptors. Therefore DHEA, like estrogen, inhibits bone resorption. (Argtielles)

3. Androgens (which includes DHEA and testosterone) stimulate bone formation and calcium absorption. DHEA might, therefore, augment the bone-building effect of progesterone. DHEA appears to be the only hormone capable of inhibiting bone resorption AND stimulating bone formation.

4. DHEA plays an important role in maintaining bone mass in postmenopausal women. In premenopausal women with Addison's disease (adrenal insufficiency), enough DHEA is apparently made by the ovaries to

compensate for the weak adrenal glands. This most likely explains why these women do not develop osteo porosis. After menopause, however, when ovarian pro duction of DHEA and other hormones slows down, the adrenal glands are not capable of taking over and a marked deficiency of DHEA results. It is quite possible that giving DHEA to postmenopausal women with adrenal insufficiency would prevent the accelerated bone loss that these women experience.

# DHEA and Calcium Metabolism

Experiments performed almost 20 years ago by Dr. Hollo, a Hungarian researcher, showed that plasma levels of DHEA-S were significantly lower in postmenopausal women with osteoporosis than in matched controls. He also found another abnormality in these women; when given calcium by intravenous injection, the calcium level in their bloodstream remained elevated for an unusually long period of time. However, after a week receiving oral DHEA-S (100 mg/day) their calcium metabolism returned to normal, suggesting that the body is making use of it. (Hollo)

Several series of data suggest that alterations in adrenal androgen output might be a contributing factor to changes in bone mass. The possible relationship between bone density and serum levels of DHEA was examined in 105 women (aged 45-69 years; 76 postmenopausal, 29 premenopausal).

Serum DHEA level was significantly lower in the individuals with low bone density. The serum DHEA level decreased significantly with age among all individuals. After correcting for age, there was a significant positive relationship between DHEA and mineral density of the bones of the lower spine, neck, and arm. Since there was no significant difference between the two groups regarding estrogens, this study suggests that DHEA may have a non-oestrogenic effect on bone. (Szathmari)

# Sex Hormones and Bone Mineral Density in Elderly Men

The relationship between sex hormones and bone mineral density in older men has been studied by a number of researchers. Testosterone is thought to play a role in determining bone mineral density in older men. (Murphy) But, there is no major correlation between osteoporosis and testosterone levels. (Buchanan, Brody) Studies have shown there is a significant correlation between bone mineralization and DHEA levels.

# Yam Cream Benefits Bone Density

Clinical studies have shown that all postmenopausal women, aged 38 to 83, using a cream with natural progesterone hormone compounds from wild yams, increased bone density levels. Some women increased their bone density levels as much as 25 percent. So, unlike estrogen, these compounds actually restore bone density. The various hormonal effects of DHEA appears to decrease bone reabsorption and increase bone formation. There were no noted side effects with this natural wild yam cream. (Lee)

The most common reason postmenopausal women take synthetic estrogen is for protection against osteoporosis. Estrogen stimulates the osteoclast bone cells to increase bone resorption. However, this effect fades after five years or so. Thereafter, bone loss continues at the same pace as in those women not using estrogen. The more important factor in osteoporosis is the lack of progesterone which causes a decrease in osteoblast-mediated new bone formation.

Patients with history of breast cancer face a future of progressive osteoporosis without recourse to hormonal therapy. These women can best benefit from natural progesterone therapy.

According to Dr. John Lee, supplemental natural progesterone derived from wild yam extract reversed their osteoporosis and, in many, it corrected their additional problems associated with the breast cancer such as vaginal atrophy. None developed cancer of any sort.

**Recommended Reading:** *"Preventing and Reversing Osteoporosis"* By Dr. Alan Gaby. Prima Publishing. P. O. Box 1260BK Rocklin, CA 95677 (916) 786-0426. In addition to information on osteoporosis, Dr. Gaby presents an excellent chapter on DHEA.

*"How to fight Osteoporosis and Win: The Miracle of Microcrystalline Hydroxyapatite"* by Beth M. Ley. BL Publications

# Chapter Summary

DHEA improves osteoporosis by increasing reabsorption and formation of bone, and by increasing the levels of other major hormones - estrogen, progesterone, and testosterone. DHEA appears to be the only hormone capable of inhibiting bone reabsorption AND stimulating bone formation.

# DHEA: THE ANTI-AGING HORMONE

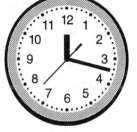

*Can DHEA turn back the time clock?*

DHEA hormone replacement therapy appears to be one of the most promising ways to slow aging while reducing the risk of degenerative diseases. DHEA could perhaps provide us with an extended lifespan, and just as important, allow us to live these years healthier, more energetic and with greater ability to do the things we like.

DHEA levels naturally go down with age as production in the adrenal glands slows. The older you are, the less DHEA you have. At age 75 or 80, women produce only 10 to 20 percent of the DHEA produced in the second decade of life. (Orentreich)

A large and rapidly expanding body of scientific evidence indicates that the level of DHEA in a person's blood can foretell the future regarding degenerative diseases such as diabetes, cancer, cardiovascular disease, memory disorders, and, perhaps, death itself.

Studies have shown a direct relationship between blood levels of DHEA and the inhibition of many diseases. DHEA has been clinically used for many years.

DHEA replacement protocol may be based upon the

objective of elevating serum DHEA levels to that of a healthy 20 to 25 year old, when levels were at their natural peak.

## *High Levels of DHEA Reduce Risk of:*

- Atherosclerosis and cardiovascular disease

- Malignant tumors and cancer

- Insulin insensitivity and diabetes

- Weight problems

- Decline in mental function and dementia, Alzheimer's, Parkinson's disease, and stroke.


These conditions are the principles associated with aging; DHEA may be the best biomarker of aging and longevity.

Cross-linking (which creates destructive, hard, inflexible bonds) is a term commonly associated with aging. Cross-linking at the molecular level causes the body to become stiff and less agile. Large protein molecules, such as collagen in connective tissue, become welded together by cross-links creating hard, inflexible arteries and wrinkled skin.

The genetic master and copy instructors of all cell functions, the nucleic acids DNA and RNA, can also be cross-linked, causing improper functioning and abnormal cells. These abnormal cells can cause aging as well as many other conditions, including cancer.

Cross-linking can be caused by a chemical, acetaldehyde, found in cigarette smoke and smog and made in the liver from alcohol; and by free radicals, destructive entities that are created by radiation and the oxidation of fats, both of which are a product of normal metabolism. Free radicals damage proteins, fats, DNA and RNA. They cause the visible brownish pigment accumulation in skin called age spots.

# Free Radicals Implicated in 60+ Diseases

Free radicals are highly reactive chemicals believed to be the cause of destruction and death in nearly all living things. Free radicals occur when healthy oxygen molecules are transformed into a highly reactive, unstable form of oxygen. This transformation occurs ironically by things we trust most like sunlight, the air we breathe, the food we eat, and things we do everyday, like exercise.

Compounded by environmental pollution, food additives, cured meats, tobacco smoke, alcohol, infection, stress, chemotherapy, asbestos, X-rays, pesticides, and other man-made pollutants, free radicals can multiply at an alarming rate.

Free radicals can attack, damage and ultimately destroy any material. They degrade collagen and reprogram DNA and are implicated in more than 60 diseases, including Alzheimer's, Parkinson's, cancer, arthritis, cataracts, kidney and liver disorders.

## *Other Areas DHEA May Benefit:*

Auto-immune diseases
   such as lupus, arthritis, allergies, asthma, etc.

Osteoporosis

Epstein-Barr

Herpes II and other viral infections

Bacterial infections

Chronic Fatigue Syndrome

AIDS

Menopause

PMS

Obesity

Emotional instability

Depression

Stress

In regard to the role of the decline of DHEA with age, we have seen that adrenalectomy can slow weight gain in young obese mice. DHEA can restore the synthesis of muscle protein to normal and lower plasma glucose. Elevated glucose levels cause insulin levels to rise. Aging, as related to hyper-insulinemia (high levels of circulating insulin which eventually cause insulin resistance by the cells), may provide insight into DHEA's functional role for preventing obesity, insulin resistance, and hyperphagia (development of abnormal cells).

The clinical decline in DHEA induced by insulin suggests that the age related decline in DHEA may be a function of increased age related insulin production. (Shimomura) However, some researchers suggest there is an opposing action between DHEA and testosterone on insulin resistance. (Buffington)

Others have postulated that aging is the result of hypo-thalamic damage resulting in hypersecretion of insulin and glucagon. (Mobbs) High insulin levels, insulin resistance, and high glucose levels all play a causative role in aging. This is in line with the concept of the age related "hyperproductive syndrome" due to the decline in DHEA.

Removal of the pituitary gland in aging mice can reverse many of the effects of aging suggesting that the neuroen-docrine system can produce a pituitary programmed death. Removal of the pituitary gland blocks collagen cross-linking in aging mice. As DHEA alters collagen metabolism, it would be of interest to see the age related effects of DHEA values without the functioning of the pituitary.


# DHEA Reduces Stress


DHEA's effect as an anti-aging hormone is partially due to its potential as a stress modulating steroid.

❏ DHEA has an adrenocortical stress-mediated blocking action.

❏ DHEA decreases the effect of liver glucocorticoid receptors.

❏ DHEA reduces shrinkage of the thymus gland.

❏ Low concentrations of DHEA to cortisol can lead to age-related stress induced central nervous system injury.

❏ Insulin induces enzyme activity (G-6-PDH) in the kidneys. DHEA may be able to reduce stress-related injury associated with changes in G-6-PDH.

❏ The antidiabetogenic action of DHEA may also relate to its ability to block corticosteroid responses. In this regard, age-related diabetes and degenerative disease may be impeded by DHEA. Whether these effects are due to ACTH or other pituitary-derived peptides has not been determined.

# DHEA Replacement in Older Individuals

Growth hormone-insulin-like growth factors (GH-IGF) decline with age in humans. Stress also reduces GH-IGF release. As levels of GH-IGF decline, muscle wasting is recognized. One question still unanswered: Does the decline of DHEA contribute to the shift from anabolism (muscle building) to muscle wasting associated with aging?

In one particular study, men and women, 40-70 years of age were given DHEA (50 mg) orally every night for six months. During each treatment period, concentrations of androgens, lipids, apolipoproteins, Growth hormone-insulin-like growth factors, insulin sensitivity, percentage of body fat, and sense of well-being were measured.

# Hormone Circulation

## Normal Activity

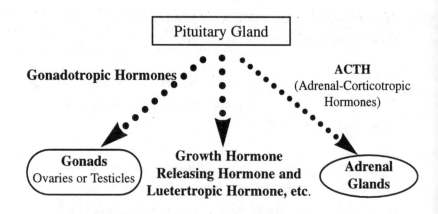

**Pituitary Gland**

**Gonadotropic Hormones**

**ACTH**
(Adrenal-Corticotropic Hormones)

**Gonads**
Ovaries or Testicles

**Growth Hormone Releasing Hormone and Luetertropic Hormone, etc.**

**Adrenal Glands**

*Balanced production distribution*

## Hormone Activity Under Stress

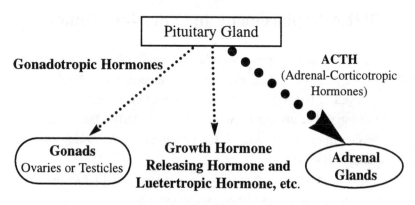

**Pituitary Gland**

**Gonadotropic Hormones**

**ACTH**
(Adrenal-Corticotropic Hormones)

**Gonads**
Ovaries or Testicles

**Growth Hormone Releasing Hormone and Luetertropic Hormone, etc.**

**Adrenal Glands**

*Unbalanced production distribution*

**The following were noted:**

❑ DHEA serum levels were restored to those found in young adults within 2 weeks of DHEA replacement and were sustained throughout the 3 months of the study.

❑ A two-fold increase in serum levels of androgens (testosterone, etc.) was observed in women, with only a small rise in androstenedione (which converts to the estrogen and testosterone sex hormones) in men.

❑ There was no change in circulating levels of sex hormone-binding globulin, estrogen, or estradiol in either gender.

❑ HDL cholesterol levels declined slightly in women, with no other lipid changes noted for either gender. Insulin  sensitivity and body fat were unaltered.

❑ Although average 24 hour growth hormone levels were unchanged, serum GF levels increased significantly, and IGF decreased significantly for both genders, suggesting an increased bioavailability of IGF to target tissues. This was associated with a remarkable increase in perceived physical and psychological well-being for both men (67 percent) and women (84 percent).

❑ The researchers concluded that improvement of physical and psychological well-being in both genders and the absence of side-effects demonstrates the novel effects of DHEA replacement in age-advanced men and women. (Morales)

# DHEA Halts Excess IL-6 Production

Aging in humans is characterized by reduced control over the production of cytokine interleukin-6 (IL-6), which is thought to play an important role in controlling abnormal cell proliferation. Increased levels of IL-6 are associated with and may contribute to many conditions associated with old age, such as cancer.

In 1993 Daynes discovered that in very old mice the immune system was secreting IL-6. Daynes demonstrated a dramatic effect of DHEA-S on excess IL-6 production. Within 24 hours of providing the DHEA-S supplement, the problem of excess production was halted. Because these measures are age related, these findings provide evidence that DHEA may help to slow normal aging. (Daynes)

## DHEA Increases Animal Lifespan by 50%

DHEA levels were found to be inversely related to death due to all causes in men over 50. (Barrett-Connor) Mice did not age as rapidly when fed DHEA, and maintained their youthful hair color and sleekness, compared with the graying, coarsening hair of the control animals. (Regelson)

## Supplemental DHEA Precautions

Although research has demonstrated that DHEA displays a broad spectrum of cancer preventive action in laboratory rodents with little toxicity, supplemental DHEA is still in the infancy stages, especially in its role as a chemotherapeutic agent. Adequate human studies have not yet been done on long-term usage of DHEA. Individuals with reproductive pre-cancerous conditions or reproductive cancers should NOT use DHEA, except under the monitoring of a health care professional.

While there is no reported toxic effects there are some reported side effects of supplemental DHEA use. Prolonged DHEA treatment with very high doses may produce some undesirable liver effects. DHEA is known to alter liver enzyme activity. (Schwartz, Leighton, Marrero)

It is very important to use antioxidants with supplemental DHEA because of this possible oxidative stress on the liver. In one rat study, vitamin E significantly reduced liver stress and was shown to have a protective effective potential of oxidative damage associated with DHEA treatment. (Schwartz, Leighton) Other studies have demonstrated the protective effect of Alpha Lipoic Acid on the liver.

In addition, because DHEA increases insulin and rate of metabolism, chromium supplementation may be a consideration. Chromium is necessary for insulin to bring glucose into the cells to be burned.

## DHEA Reverses Aging

Preliminary results in mice suggest that DHEA may retard the aging process. Animals treated with this hormone looked younger, had glossier coats, and less gray hair than control animals.

In humans, serum levels of DHEA are known to decline with age. The levels in seventy-year-old individuals are only about 20 percent as high as those in young adults. This age-related decline is not known to occur with any other adrenal steroids. It has, therefore, been suggested that many of the manifestations of aging may be caused by DHEA deficiency. In my experience, some elderly people who suffer from weakness, muscle wasting, tremulousness, and other signs of aging experience noticeable improvements within several weeks of beginning small doses of DHEA (5-15 mg/day).

Research shows that due to age-related changes in metabolism (the conversion of food to energy) the daily requirements of a number of important nutrients increase. Some authorities tell us that the present RDAs may actually result in insufficiencies of certain nutrients leading to increased risk of later stage diseases.

Many old-age diseases are actually the consequence of suboptimal nutrition over time which increased the risk for these conditions later in life.

We know that specific nutrients, vitamins B-6, B-12, C,

D, and E and the minerals calcium, zinc, iron, and chromium, are required in significantly larger amounts as we grow older to optimize function.

The U.S. Surgeon General estimates that two-thirds of the illnesses suffered in old age are preventable. At the top of the list as negative contributors for those who died earliest in the study were sedentary lifestyle and smoking, neither of which has a positive effect on DHEA levels.

Overall, the study showed that good habits could promote an advantage in health of 30 years over those who had bad habits. The major conclusion of the UCLA study: A balanced lifestyle is one of the most important steps toward retarding the aging process.

America seems to fixate on being young forever. Young, beautiful bodies fill the pages of magazines and television and movie screens. To those who know the U.S. only by advertising or television, it is a paradise inhabited by beautiful, shapely people under 30. But the image of the U.S. as the land of eternal youth is grossly at odds with reality. The majority of people are over age 50 and the number of people reaching senior status is growing faster than any other age group.

## Chapter Summary

DHEA levels decrease with age. At the age of 75 or 80, we produce only 10 to 20 percent of the DHEA produced in the second decade of life. DHEA levels can foretell our future regarding degenerative diseases such as diabetes, cancer, cardiovascular disease, memory disorders, and perhaps death itself. There is a direct relationship between blood levels of DHEA and the inhibition of many diseases. DHEA has been clinically used for anti-aging and for therapeutic purposes for many years.

# DHEA AND AGING

*Special Segment by Dr. Samuel S. C. Yen*

*Following are the preliminary results of the 1993-1994 DHEA and Aging trial conducted by Dr. Samuel S. C. Yen, M.D., W. R. Persons Professor of Reproductive Medicine, UCSD School of Medicine and Medical Center, San Diego, CA., presented at the DHEA and Aging meeting sponsored by the New York Academy of Sciences on June 18, 1995 in Washington, D.C.*

Summary: *"Our preliminary results using DHEA replacement in well- controlled human trials suggest that DHEA replacement has both psychological and physiological benefits for the aging population. DHEA replacement may, at a future date, be applicable for clinical use in the aging population."* **Dr. Samuel S. C. Yen**

## Most Recent DHEA Replacement Study

In 1993, a double-blind, placebo controlled one-year study was initiated which involved eight men and eight women over age 50. Each patient took either a 100 mg dose of DHEA or a placebo for the first six months, and then crossed-over to take the opposite for the second six months. The goal of this study was to measure DHEA's effects on several biological end-points.

**Preliminary results of the 1993/1994 trial include:**

● DHEA blood levels were restored to those found in young adults within two weeks of DHEA replacement.

115

● Blood levels of IGF-I (insulin-like growth factor) increased significantly in both women and men. This growth factor declines with age and has a multifunctional role in the regulation of cell metabolism and the immune system; thus, it helps regulate cellular well-being.

● Muscle mass and muscle strength increased for both men and women. Men experienced only a slight decline in body fat.

● Immune function in men improved, with a significant increase in function of natural killer cells (immune system cells that fight viruses) and interleukin-2 secretion. Effects on immune system function in women are being analyzed.

### No Change

● Insulin sensitivity, which is involved in diabetes, did not change. There was also no change in lipids.

● There was no change in libido.

### Study History: DHEA Replacement

● In 1985, Dr. Yen began studying the mechanism of DHEA decline in aging women. Yen's group found that an enzyme (17,20 desmolase) essential for synthesis of DHEA is functionally reduced with aging. Since it was not possible to activate or replace the enzyme, Yen turned to "replacement therapy" for DHEA. To determine the right dose, Yen conducted a pharmacokinetics study in postmenopausal women.

These studies led to the formulation of a 50 mg daily replacement dose of DHEA. This is a synthetic powder form of DHEA in a capsule to be taken orally before bedtime. Levels of DHEA in the body naturally increase at night.

● In 1990, a six-month, double-blind, placebo controlled

study was conducted with 13 men and 17 women, aged 40 to 70. Each patient took either a 50 mg dose of DHEA or a placebo for the first three months, and then crossed-over to take the opposite for the second three months. The researchers measured levels of the growth factor IGF-I. The results of this study were published in the June 1994 issue of the *Journal of Clinical Endocrinology and Metabolism.*

**Results of 1990 Study:**

● Biochemical change (as measured in the lab from blood samples)

● Increased IGF-I (insulin growth factor). This growth factor declines with age and has a multifunctional role in the regulation of cell metabolism and the immune system; thus, it helps regulate cellular well-being.

● Perceived sense of well-being: At the end of each three-month treatment arm, volunteers were given questionnaires about their feelings of overall well-being. A majority of the participants, 67 percent of men and 84 percent of women, reported an increased sense of well-being after taking DHEA. After taking the placebo, less than 10 percent of men and women reported an increased sense of well-being.

In an open-ended questionnaire, patients reported:
● Increased ability to cope with stress
● Increased physical mobility
● Improved quality of sleep
● Decreased joint pain

**Definition of DHEA:**

● DHEA is a quasi-steroid hormone secreted by the adrenal gland in amounts exceeding all other steroid hormones by the endocrine glands.

● DHEA secretion increases dramatically at the time of early puberty, reaching a peak at ages 25 to 30. DHEA has been called a "marker" of aging because after age 30 it declines progressively to 10 percent of young adult levels by age 70. Apart from inducing early pubertal development, the biological function of DHEA is elusive. Animal studies suggest DHEA has numerous protective effects in body function and diseases. It is a multifunctional hormone with an important role in the regulation of the immune system and general cellular "well-being."

*Dr. Yen's collaborators at UCSD School of Medicine: Omid Khorram, M.D., Arlene Morales, M.D., John Nolan, M.D., Jerry Nelson, M.D.*

*For more information you may contact the Sam and Rose Stein Institute For Research On Aging University of California, San Diego School of Medicine, 9500 Gilman Drive, La Jolla, CA 92093-0664  Phone 619-534-6299 Fax 619-534-5475. Yearly memberships start at just $30.00.*

Dr. Samuel Yen has been involved in numerous aging and hormone studies. He, along with Drs. AJ Morales, JJ Nolan, and JC Nelson, from the Department of Reproductive Medicine, University of California School of Medicine in La Jolla, published their results on the "Effects of replacement dose of dehydroepiandrosterone in men and women of advancing age" in the *Journal of Clinical Endocrinological Metabolism* in June 1994. The summary of these results follows:

Aging in humans is accompanied by a progressive decline in the secretion of the adrenal androgens dehydroepiandrosterone (DHEA) and DHEA sulfate (DHEA-S), paralleling that of the GH-insulin-like growth factor. Although the functional relationship of the decline of the GH-IGF-I system and catabolism (muscle wasting) is recognized, the biological role of DHEA in human aging remains undefined. To test the hypothesis that the decline in DHEA may contribute to the shift from anabolism to catabolism associated with aging, the effect of a replacement dose of DHEA in 13 men and 17 women, 40-70 years of age was studied.

A randomized placebo-controlled cross-over trial of nightly oral DHEA administration (50 mg) of 6-month duration was conducted. During each treatment period, concentrations of androgens, lipids, apolipoproteins, IGF-I, IGF-binding protein-1 (IGFBP-1), IGFBP-3, insulin sensitivity, percent body fat, libido, and sense of well-being were measured.

A subgroup of men and women underwent 24-h sampling at 20-minute intervals for GH determinations. DHEA and DHEA-S serum levels were restored to those found in young adults within 2 weeks of DHEA replacement and were sustained throughout the 3 months of the study.

A 2-fold increase in serum levels of androgens (androstenedione, testosterone, and dihydrotestosterone) was observed in women, with only a small rise in androstenedione (which converts to the estrogen and testosterone sex hormones) in men. There was no change in circulating levels of sex hormone-binding globulin, estrone, or estradiol in either gender. High density lipoprotein levels declined slightly in women, with no other lipid changes noted for either gender. Insulin sensitivity and percent body fat were unaltered. Although mean 24-h GH and IGFBP-3 levels were unchanged, serum IGF-I levels increased significantly, and IGFBP-1 decreased significantly for both genders, suggesting an increased bioavailability of IGF-I to target tissues.

119

This was associated with a remarkable increase in perceived physical and psychological well-being for both men (67%) and women (84%) and no change in libido.

In conclusion, restoring DHEA and DHEA-S to young adult levels in men and women of advancing age induced an increase in the bioavailability of IGF-I, as reflected by an increase in IGF-I and a decrease in IGFBP-1 levels. These observations together with improvement of physical and psychological well-being in both genders and the absence of side-effects constitute the first demonstration of novel effects of DHEA replacement in age-advanced men and women.

In another hormone related study, Dr. Samuel Yen with Drs A.A. Murphy, L.M. Kettel, A.J. Morales, and V.J. Roberts, also from the University of California, San Diego School of Medicine, reported on the effects of the antiprogesterone RU486 in the *Journal of Clinical Endocrinological Metabolism,* February 1993. They describe how RU 486 has regressionary effects on steroid hormone dependent fibroid tumors by withdrawal of progesterone action and/or by its interference of estrogen action. They also noted that RU486 caused a significant rise in serum DHEA-S and cortisol, suggesting an antiglucocorticoid effect of RU486.

The same group also reported that RU 486 can improve symptoms and growth of pelvic endometriosis. This was published in *Fertility and Sterility,* 1993.

*This information is used by permission granted from Dr. Samuel Yen in a phone conversation 11/10/95.*

# DHEA AND SEX

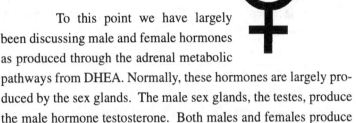

To this point we have largely been discussing male and female hormones as produced through the adrenal metabolic pathways from DHEA. Normally, these hormones are largely produced by the sex glands. The male sex glands, the testes, produce the male hormone testosterone. Both males and females produce this hormone, but males produce more than females.

Ovaries, the female sex gland, produce estrogen and progesterone. Males also produce these hormones in minute amounts. All of our glands work in relation to one another. Without estrogen, certain glands cannot function well, but with too much estrogen other glands may be disturbed. Estrogen can step up the growth of abnormal cancer cells. Birth control pills, which contain estrogen, may be incompatible with your health history, especially if you have had a liver tumor or breast cancer. Diabetics, smokers, women who have used birth control pills, have cardiovascular problems, high blood pressure, elevated cholesterol levels, or who have a family history of early cardiovascular trouble, might risk their health by taking estrogen.

In 1968 the low-dose estrogen birth control pill was introduced. It has helped to reduce the number of blood clots in the veins of women, but has had no effect on artery disease or the overall death rate. In other words, women on the low-dose pill are still at an increased risk of dying from circulatory disease.

In *The Lancet,* the Royal College of General

121

Practitioners revealed that women who have used the pill have a 40 percent higher death rate, mostly from circulatory disease.

Despite reports that the pill protects against breast cancer, there are more deaths from breast cancer among women on the pill than not on the pill. If you smoke and take the pill, there is a stronger chance that you will get cardiovascular disease. Both smoking and birth control pills suppress natural hormone production and functions. After years of this insult to the body many women with menopause, experience further insult through hormone replacement therapy. Estrogen analogs further insult an even more vulnerable age group.

All hormones secreted by the endocrine glands serve to regulate balance of the body chemistry, and to maintain homeostasis. Under normal circumstances the chemical makeup of our blood fluctuates within a narrow range. The blood glucose level rises and falls a little. The amount of calcium in the blood goes up and down very slightly. All of the different chemicals in the body fluctuate within a very narrow range when the body is healthy. The minerals, enzymes, and hormones in the bloodstream can work together only when the body mechanisms are working correctly to maintain homeostasis.

## Stress and Sex

Stress and sex don't mix. During stress the sex glands, the ovaries and testes, shrink and become less active. This is in proportion to the enlargement and increased activity of the adrenals. The sex glands are stimulated by gonadotropin hormones which are stimulated by the pituitary glands. *(See page 94)* In times of stress the pituitary gland has to put out greater amounts of ATCH which stimulates the adrenal glands. This requires so much effort from the pituitary that it must reduce its output of other "less important" hormones such as the gonadotropin hormones. Stress affects the production of milk in lactating females and can cause irregular menstruation. Premenstrual syndrome has been associated with this adaptive response to stress.

In men, stress can cause both the diminishment of the sexual urge and sperm cell production.

# DHEA and Libido

Most of our sex hormones are derived from enzymes acting on DHEA. So technically speaking, without DHEA, one would think that the levels of these other hormones would be greatly diminished as well, and without these hormones, we have no sex drive. This does not hold true entirely because the ovaries and testicles, in good health do produce sex hormones as well. But, when they don't, DHEA from the adrenal glands is supposed to pick up the slack.

Scientists presently are experimenting with supplemental DHEA to confirm earlier studies that demonstrate DHEA's ability to improve sex drive, increase fertility and other problems associated with decreased sex hormones which accompanies aging. A number of men have reported a dramatic change in their sex drive stating that their libido was what they had in their 20's after taking DHEA. *(See Appendix I)* To date, no published studies, including the Samuel Yen study at the University of California School of Medicine, have reported any change in libido among men. (Morales, Yen ) *See pages 141-143, and 166.*

One study in 1984 by the Crenshaw Clinic has demonstrated a favorable association between women's sex drives and DHEA.

Pheromones, our sexual scent, is derived from DHEA. Pheromones dictate sexual behavior among animals. This smell is also involved in bonding between babies and their mothers after birth.

# Male Reproductive System

Sperm and male sex hormones are produced in the testes. Sperm travels from each testes into the epididymis, along coiled tubes where they mature and are stored.

## Puberty

Male sexual capability, or virility, begins at puberty. Puberty occurs when secondary sexual characteristics appear and sexual organs mature, allowing reproduction to take place. Physical and emotional changes characterize puberty and adolescence, around age 12 and 15. It is initiated by pituitary hormones (gonadotropins) which stimulates development of the testes and production and secretion of androgens such as testosterone. Secondary sexual characteristics, such as the appearance of pubic, underarm and facial hair, also occur. Testosterone stimulates the production of sperm and causes the seminal vesicles and prostate gland to mature. Testosterone is responsible for the characteristic growth and distribution of hair on face, chest and abdomen, the pitch of the voice, and the width of the shoulders.

## Androgens

The hormones associated with male characteristics (facial and body hair, decreased body fat, musculature, muscle strength, etc.) are called androgens. Androgens have an anabolic effect by increasing the rate of protein synthesis. This accelerates growth and increases muscle size. Androgens are also responsible for the typical male aggressive behavior. Acne, due to an accumulation of excessive sebum, results from androgen production. These hormones may also be responsible for male-pattern baldness.

Since the adrenal glands also secrete androgens in both sexes, manipulation of this process in women through drug therapy can result in the development of the secondary sexual characteristics of men, as well as amenorrhea (absence of menstruation in women). Abuses of this process are most often seen among athletes who take androgens.

## Testosterone

Testosterone is the main male androgen. It is produced in the male testicles and also through the adrenal metabolic pathways in both men and women. Women produce far less quantities of testosterone compared to males.

## Male Menopause (Andropause)

Male menopause, associated with male aging, coincides with progressive impairment of testicular function, largely the production of testosterone. The symptom associated with male menopause include loss of sex drive, depression, anxiety, calcium loss increasing the risk for the development of osteoporosis, decreased musculature, increased fat storage, decreased insulin sensitivity, and negative effects on the central nervous system.

In healthy individuals, bioavailable testosterone declines by approximately one percent per year between ages 40 and 70, but a more pronounced decline has been observed in nonhealthy groups, especially in high cardiovascular risk groups. Androgen (testosterone) deficiency might be treated by an appropriate androgen supplementation.

## The Prostate

The prostate is a small chestnut-shaped organ that surrounds the neck of the bladder and the upper part of the urethra. The prostate gland consists of an inner zone which produces secretions that help moisten the urethra, and an outer zone in which seminal secretions are produced. This substance makes semen into a liquid. The seminal vesicles pass through the prostate to enter the urethra. Under the influence of androgens at puberty, the prostate begins to mature, reaching full size and weight by about age 20.

The normal aging process in men leads to the development of Benign Prostate Hypertrophy (BPH), often referred to as an enlarged prostate, due to a variety of factors, including age-related alterations in hormone levels.

As men age there are many significant changes in hormone levels. Testosterone and free testosterone levels decrease after age 50, while other hormones - prolactin, oestradiol, sex hormone-binding ligand, luteinizing hormone and follicle stimulating hormone levels all increase. The effect of these changes is an increased concentration of testosterone within the prostate. This testosterone is responsible for the overproduction of prostate cells which result in prostatic enlargement.

The increase of testosterone within the prostatic cell is largely due to a decreased rate of removal. Testosterone is normally metabolized by enzymes to compounds that have a reduced attraction for receptor molecules in the cells that bind these hormones. The metabolized testosterone is then excreted. Since the hormones are not being metabolized and excreted, levels of the hormones increase within the prostatic cells. Elevated estrogen levels play a role in the development of BPH by inhibiting the enzymes that metabolize testosterone.

In addition to a decreased rate of excretion of the male hormones by the prostate in BPH, there is also an increase in the uptake of testosterone by the prostate. This appears to be the result of yet another hormone, prolactin, which increases the uptake of testosterone and increases the synthesis of another type of testosterone, dihydrotestosterone. The net result is that the more potent androgen, dihydrotestosterone is greatly increased within the prostate in BPH.

Prolactin levels are increased by beer consumption and stress. These factors may contribute greatly to BPH. Drugs that reduce prolactin levels reduce many of the symptoms of BPH. However, these drugs have severe side effects and are therefore not widely used.

It appears that the trace mineral zinc and vitamin B6 can reduce prolactin levels, without any side effects at prescribed doses. As zinc and vitamin B6 are intricately involved in hormone metabolism, deficiency of one or both of these nutrients may be a contributing factor in the cause of BPH in many men.

# Prostate Cancer

Cancer of the prostate is the second most common malignancy in men. After lung and colon cancers it ranks as the third most common cause of cancer death in all men over the age of 55. Prostate cancer accounts for about 19 percent of all male cancers in the U.S. In different parts of the world, its frequency varies with the amount of dietary saturated fat. The U.S. has 14 deaths per 100,000 men per year from prostate cancer. Sweden has 22 deaths, and Japan has only two deaths per 100,000 men.

# Sexual Function Declines With Age in Men

Sexual function, and in particular erectile capacity, declines with age in men. (Rowland) Unlike women, fertility in men persists until a very old age. However, testicular function decreases in old age, causing symptoms which are analogous to, although less pronounced than, the menopausal syndrome. These symptoms can be considered male andropause.

However, at menopause ovarian hormonal secretion ceases almost completely, but the decrease in the levels of biologically active free testosterone is only moderate. Many elderly men actually have free androgen levels that would be considered normal for young men.

Exercise, for example, increases androgen levels in both men and women. Individuals who exercise on a regular basis report better overall health and seem to age much slower compared to those who do not exercise on a regular basis.

Many well-controlled studies have shown the benefit of hormonal replacement therapy, at least for symptomatic post-menopausal women, but, so far, no well-controlled studies exist that prove a favorable risk/benefit balance of androgen substitution in elderly men. The major risk is the potentially stimulating effect of androgens in elderly men who are at risk for prostate cancer. (Vermeulen)

## Male Stroke Patients Experience Low Levels of Testosterone

Low levels of serum insulin-like growth factor-I (IGF-I) and testosterone were found among men with post-stroke paralysis. Serum concentrations of IGF-I, and testosterone were compared in healthy young men, healthy old men, and in old men with post-stroke paralysis.

Low IGF-I levels were found in 85 percent of the healthy old men, and in 88 percent of the post-stroke paralysis patients. The prevalence in the men with paralysis was only five percent of normal healthy levels.

For testosterone, a value below the lower 2.5 percentile in the healthy young men, occurred in 78 percent of the healthy old men and in 79 percent of the stroke survivors. Low testosterone occurred in 17 percent of the men with paralysis.

Compared with healthy young men, most healthy old men have low serum IGF-I and testosterone levels. Old men with paralysis resemble healthy old men in their IGF-I levels, but they have more cases of severe hypogonadism (low testosterone). Because correction of IGF-I and testosterone deficiencies in younger adults improves muscle strength, work capacity, and quality of life, treatment with human growth hormone and testosterone may be a useful adjunct to physical measures in the rehabilitation of selected stroke survivors. (Abbasi)

# Supplemental Testosterone

Supplemental testosterone is given to women for female breast cancer and to men and women for growth stimulation, muscular development, and red blood cell production. Testosterone given to correct deficiencies in young adults improves muscle strength, work capacity, and quality of life. (Abbasi) Hormone studies conducted on strength development in middle-aged to elderly males and females showed that testosterone supplementation increased leg strength in both men and women. (Hakkinen)

Serious side effects include fluid retention, masculization in women including unnatural hair growth and deep voice, acne, a blood disease called erythrocythemia, prostate enlargement causing urinary retention, and high blood pressure or heart disease.

In men, prolonged use of synthetic steroid hormones can reduce sperm count and volume of semen, cause atrophy of the testicles, and possibly cause kidney stones, and leukemia. The potential increased risk for development of prostate cancer has been the main reason for limiting indications of such treatment. A 1.8 year survey of men aged 55-70 years treated with testosterone suggested that high plasma levels of testosterone effectively induced clinical benefits while reducing prostate size. (de Lignieres)

Effective testosterone treatment of hypogonadal men results in prostate volume and prostate-specific antigen levels comparable to age-matched normal men. Therefore, testosterone-induced prostate growth should not inhibit hypogonadal men from testosterone substitution therapy. (Behre)

# Replacement Therapy Reduces Health Risks

Individuals with adult-onset growth hormone deficiency, which also occurs with aging, have an increased risk for cardiovascular disease. Individuals using replacement therapy (RT) were studied to determine whether the replacement therapy had a beneficial effect upon their risk for cardiovascular disease. They found:

❑ The RT patients had a significantly higher body mass index (lower body fat) compared to controls.

❑ The RT patients had higher triglyceride levels but their was no difference in total serum cholesterol concentration. Serum high-density lipoprotein (HDL) cholesterol was lower in RT patients.
❑ There was no difference in the prevalence of diabetes mellitus.

❑ The prevalence of treated hypertension was higher in the patients but the prevalence of smoking was lower.

Even after taking the increased body mass index into consideration, the changes in the prevalence of treated hypertension and in the serum concentrations of triglycerides and high-density lipoprotein concentrations remained. This shows that growth hormone deficiency alters fat metabolism and increases the risk for development of hypertension, which contributes to the increased risk for cardiovascular disease. (Rosen)

## High Testosterone and DHEA Levels Mean Elevated Insulin Levels in Men, but not Women

Many studies indicate that increased levels of male-associated hormones are associated with insulin resistance and hyper-insulinemia in both premenopausal and postmenopausal women, but this is not the case for men. In a study group of 178 men, after adjustment for age, obesity, and body fat distribution, insulin concentrations were significantly inversely correlated with testosterone and DHEA. This is in striking contrast to women, where increased androgenicity is associated with insulin resistance and high insulin levels. (Haffner)

# The Female Reproductive System

The sex hormones, such as estrogen and progesterone, which control the reproductive or menstrual cycle, are secreted from the ovaries and are produced through the endocrine pathways as well as through the adrenals via DHEA.

## Estrogen and Progesterone

These are the two main groups of hormones essential for normal sexual development and healthy functioning of the reproductive system. Estrogens play an important role in the total health of women throughout life. Estrogens are produced mainly in the ovaries, but to some degree in the adrenals. During pregnancy, they may also be produced in the placenta.

Progesterone increases the deposition of fats and increases the production of sebum in the glands of the skin which can cause acne.

Progesterone, produced in the ovaries, is also an important hormone for the health of the female reproductive system. It is produced during the second half of the menstrual cycle, and by the placenta during pregnancy. Following ovulation, progesterone levels increase and cause endometrium (the lining of the uterus) to thicken in preparation for receiving a fertilized ovum. Should fertilization not occur the production of progesterone and estrogen decreases and the endometrium is shed along with the unfertilized egg during menstruation.

Progesterone assures that a fetus develops in a healthy manner by maintaining the health of the placenta. The natural drop in progesterone at the end of pregnancy helps initiate labor.

## Menstruation

Menstruation refers to the cycle shedding of the endometrium or uterus lining.  It is indicated by bleeding.  Menstruation occurs during the fertile years of a woman's life (puberty to menopause).  When the body stops producing eggs, menstruation ceases.

Menstruation is under the control of hormones, estrogen during the first part of the cycle, and progesterone during the second half.  Other hormones regulate other parts of the menstrual cycle.

Mature eggs from the ovaries enter the fallopian tubes following ovulation.  Ovulation refers to the development and release of an ovum from a follicle halfway through the menstrual cycle.  Follicle stimulating hormone (FSH) is responsible for stimulating the growth of the egg during the first half of the cycle.  Then luteinizing hormone (LH) stimulates the release of just one ovum (normally).  The follicle forms a mass of tissue called the corpus luteum that secretes progesterone during the second half of the cycle.

Once the ovum enters the fallopian tube it travels along until met by a sperm traveling up the tube from the uterus.  If there is no sperm present at that time, the ovum is shed during menstruation.

## Premenstrual Syndrome (PMS)

PMS involves the physical and emotional symptoms many women experience during the week or two before menstruation.  It usually begins in conjunction with ovulation and continues until the onset of menstruation.  Many women experience changes such as irritability, depression, mood swings, food cravings, backache, and headache, all of which may be severe enough to interfere with daily life.

The cause of the symptoms are directly related to hormonal changes, specifically, the production of progesterone and luteinizing hormone (LH). The ovaries produce progesterone in the second half of the menstrual cycle. Luteinizing hormone is produced in the pituitary in the brain and controls ovulation and a specific antibody. Women with PMS have a significantly lower level of circulating LH antibody compared to women without symptoms.

Natural progesterone directly stimulated circulating LH is believed to control the symptoms of PMS. Supplemental DHEA increases progesterone as does diosgenin extracted from wild yam. (Lee)

### *90 percent of all women experience one or more of the reported symptoms of PMS.*

| | |
|---|---|
| Anxiety | Irritability |
| Mood swings | Tension |
| Bloating | Breast tenderness |
| Fluid retention | Weight gain |
| Cravings for sweets | Dizziness |
| Fatigue | Headache |
| Increased appetite | Heart palpitations |
| Confusions | Crying |
| Depression | Forgetfulness |
| Insomnia | Withdrawal |

Dr. John Lee, M.D., points out that the symptoms of PMS and the side effects of estrogen are remarkably similar. Though not completely understood, PMS seems to represent an individual reaction to estrogen dominance secondary to a relative progesterone deficiency. This hormone imbalance is believed to be the result of stress, nutritional deficiencies, high fat diet, and the use (past or present) of synthetic contraceptive pills.

Dr. Lee has found success using natural progesterone from wild yam extract administered transdermally in his practice for patients experiencing symptoms of PMS. He states,

*"The results were most impressive. The majority (but not all) of such patients reported remarkable improvement in their symptom-complex, including the elimination of their premenstrual water retention and weight gain."*

# Menopause

This term refers to the cessation of menstruation as a result of slowed estrogen production. It includes a sometimes lengthy period of time, beginning between the ages of 45 and 55, when menstruation becomes irregular and the production of female sex hormones goes through periodic fluctuations in intensity and quality.

Eventually, the follicles cease to produce eggs, which leads to a decrease in estrogen production. Without the influence of estrogen, an increase in the level of gonodotropin hormones and androgens may occur.

More than half of menopausal women experience hot flashes and night sweats. These symptoms may last up to five or more years. Over 20 percent experience significant vaginal dryness. In all women, the vagina itself will shrink and lose elasticity and become more susceptible to infection. The breasts sag and the skin will lose its softness. The result might be a variety of unsettling physiological and psychological symptoms:

| | |
|---|---|
| Hot flashes | Vaginal dryness |
| Osteoporosis | Heart palpitations |
| Panic attacks | Night sweats |
| Dry and burning eyes | Depression |
| Migraines, etc. | |

One of the most troublesome aspects of menopause is the loss of calcium from the bones. Over time this can lead to severe osteoporosis. Menopause may also produce an increased risk of hypertension and elevated blood cholesterol levels which may, in turn, produce atherosclerosis, and increase the risk of stroke or coronary heart disease.

# Progesterone and Menopause

Hormone therapy using synthetic progesterone or progestins and synthetic estrogen (which is made from the urine of pregnant horses), is widely prescribed for menopausal therapy.

In spite of all of the known side effects and risks associated with taking these synthetic analogs, most doctors continue to prescribe them. Instead of helping, these synthetic analogs often aggravate symptoms causing irritability and emotional problems. While estrogen has shown to have beneficial cardiovascular effects, progestins exerts a detrimental effect on blood lipids by increasing LDL and reducing HDL cholesterol.

### *Potential Side Effects of Synthetic Progesterone*

| | |
|---|---|
| Uterine / Breast cancer | Blood clots |
| Fluid retention / Swelling | Breast tenderness |
| Weight gain | Depression |
| Skin breakouts / Acne | Alopecia (hair loss) |
| Breakthrough bleeding | Masculizing effects, |
| Spotting | i.e., excess body hair |
| Amenorrhea | Changes in libido |
| Nausea | Dizziness |
| Insomnia | Sleepiness |
| Acute allergic reaction | Pulmonary embolism |
| Mental depression | Rise in blood pressure |
| Decreased glucose tolerance | Migraine headaches |
| Nervousness | |

With the onset of menopause women experience the increased risk for development of osteoporosis. For years synthetic hormones have been recommended. But, John Lee, M.D., in his 1993 book, *Natural Progesterone*, states that not only can natural progesterone serve as a prevention for osteoporosis, it can actually reverse it. He used transdermal application of wild Mexican yam extract and proved that osteoporosis is reversible in almost 100 percent of the cases he followed. This was without the use of dangerous synthetic estrogens that increase the risk of breast, endometrial cancers, and other diseases.

## Hormone Replacement Therapy

Many women resort to hormone replacement therapy with synthetic estrogens to help counteract menopausal changes. The side effects from these drugs can be very unpleasant. Breast tenderness, bloating, weight gain, nausea, reduced sex drive, depression, headaches, and vaginal bleeding are common. They also increase risk for blood clots which could precipitate stroke and increase hypertension.

In menopause, progesterone drugs are usually combined with estrogen drugs to reduce the risk of cancer of the uterus from the estrogens. But progesterone drugs themselves have unpleasant side effects, including headache, swelling, weight gain, loss of appetite, dizziness blackouts, risk, irregular periods, breast tenderness, and ovarian cysts.

Many postmenopausal women do not need estrogen supplements. Not only does a woman's body continue to produce some estrogen but she is ingesting phytoestrogens (estrogenic substances found in plants) and is exposed to xenoestrogens (environmental estrogenic substances of petrochemical origin). The addition of progesterone enhances the receptors of estrogen and thus her need for estrogen may not exist.

Hot flashes are not a sign of estrogen deficiency, but are

due to heightened hypothalamic activity due to low levels of progesterone and estrogen. If these levels were raised, a negative feedback message is sent to the pituitary and hypothalamus. Once progesterone levels are raised, estrogen receptors become more sensitive, and hot flashes usually subside.

# Estrogens

There is no specific hormone named estrogen. Estrogen is the name for a class of female steroid hormone compounds of which there are 20 or so members. The major estrogens are estrone (E-1), estradiol (E-2), and estriol (E-3).

Estrogens aid the development of secondary female sex traits such as breast development and fat deposited under the skin. Estrogen deficiency and amenorrhea (absence of monthly menstrual flow) have many causes including prolactin-producing tumors, anorexia nervosa, intense exercise associated with leanness, as well as natural or surgical menopause.

Estrogens are associated with procreation and survival of the fetus, as it is advantageous to the baby for the expectant mother to be able, in times of famine, to store body fat. Thus, the effects of estrogen include far more than merely its action on creating a shapely female body and its stimulation of the uterus and breasts. During times of consistent dietary abundance (especially excess fat in the diet), estrogen's effects are potentially undesirable.

### Estrogen Effects

Creates proliferative endometrium

Stimulates breasts

Increases body fat

Causes salt and fluid retention

Causes depression and headaches

137

Interferes with thyroid hormone

Increases blood clotting

Decreases libido

Impairs blood sugar control

Causes loss of zinc and retention of copper

Reduces oxygen levels in all cells

Increases risk of endometrial cancer

Increases risk of breast cancer

Slightly restrains osteoclast function

Reduces vascular tone

# Potential Risks of Synthetic Estrogen

Supplemental estrogen is used in oral contraceptives to treat postmenopausal breast cancer and prostate cancer and to inhibit the production of breast milk. It is also used to prevent miscarriage, and treat osteoporosis and ovarian disease.

Although many physicians recommend estrogen replacement for postmenopausal women, it is generally agreed that the detrimental health risks outweighs the benefit in most women at risk for osteoporosis.

Ads for Premarin™ brand of conjugated estrogen tablets can be found in many women's and health magazines. They market to women concerned about osteoporosis and menopause. Premarin™ is described as a complex blend of estrogens manufactured by a 125-step, 6-week process. Something that requires so much processing seems far from anything natural and beneficial to the body.

## *Potential Side Effects of Premarin*™

Increased risk for cancer of the breast and uterus

Gall bladder disease

Abnormal blood clotting

Heart disease

Excessively high calcium levels

Nausea, vomiting, cramps

Yellowing of the skin and/or whites of eyes

Breast tenderness or enlargement

Enlargement of benign tumors of the uterus

Breakthrough bleeding or spotting

Vaginal yeast infections

Fluid retention (This can make some heath conditions worse such as epilepsy, migraine headaches, heart disease and kidney disease)

Skin rashes, darkening or reddening of the skin, especially the face

Headaches, dizziness, faintness or changes in vision (including intolerance to contact lens)

Mental depression

Asthma (increase in severity)

Hair loss or abnormal hairiness

Increase or decrease in weight

Change in sex drive

Blood sugar instability

Many of estrogen's undesirable side effects are effectively prevented by progesterone. It is the custom of contemporary medicine to prescribe estrogen alone for women without intact uteri and, equally unfortunate, premenopausal estrogen dominance is simply ignored.

During the 1970's it became obvious that post-menopausal women taking unopposed estrogen for hot flashes, prevention of osteoporosis, etc., were at increased risk of endometrial cancer. This type of cancer is an uncommon occurrence before menopause when one has normal levels of estrogen and progesterone. Combined hormone therapy (using both estrogen and a progestin) in postmenopausal women can reduce the risk of estrogen-induced endometrial cancer.

Remember that there are many additional hormones in the body besides estrogens and progesterone. Any time a synthetic hormone is introduced to the body, the hormonal balance of the body is upset. Problems, which are referred to as side effects, are then the result of this imbalance. One can attempt to balance estrogen and progesterone, helping to eliminate some potential problems, but there are dozens of other hormones to also be concerned with. The bottom line is once you start messing with the hormonal balance of the body by introducing a synthetic, you cannot avoid side effects.

## Estrogen and Breast Cancer

Not all estrogens are equivalent in their actions on breast tissue. Among the three major natural estrogens, estradiol is the most stimulating to breast tissue, estrone is second, and estriol by far the least. During pregnancy, estriol is the dominant estrogen, being produced in great quantities by the placenta while ovarian production of estradiol and estrone is quiescent. Since all estrogens compete for the same receptor sites, it is probable that sufficient estriol reduces the carcinogenic effects of estradiol and/or estrone.

Estrogen is somehow related to the development of breast cancer. The cancer protective benefit of progesterone is clearly indicated by the prospective study in which pre-menopausal women with low progesterone levels were found to have many times the risk of developing premenopausal breast cancer and a ten fold increase in deaths from all malignant tumors compared to those with normal progesterone levels.

Almost 30 years ago, it was reported that women with breast cancer excreted 30-60 percent less estriol than non-cancer controls and that remission of cancer in patients receiving endocrine therapy occurred on in those whose estriol level rose. That is, low levels of estriol relative to estradiol and estrone correlate with increased risk of breast cancer and higher levels of estriol from endocrine treatment correlate with remission of cancer. (Lemmon)

Thus, the evidence is strong that unopposed estradiol and estrone are carcinogenic for breasts, and both progesterone and estriol, the two major hormones throughout pregnancy, are protective against breast cancer. These two beneficial and safe hormones could be used for women whenever hormone supplementation is indicated. Both hormones are available and are relatively inexpensive. Why have these two hormones been neglected by contemporary medical practice in favor of synthetic analog substitutes?

## Estrogen and Endometrial Cancer

It is generally acknowledged that the only known cause of endometrial cancer is unopposed estrogen, specifically, estradiol and estrone. When given to postmenopausal women for five years it increases the risk of endometrial cancer six fold. Longer use increases the risk to 15-fold. In premenopausal women, endometrial cancer is extremely rare except during the 5-10 years before menopause when estrogen dominance is common. The addition of natural progesterone during these years would significantly reduce the incidence of endometrial cancer (as well as breast cancer).

Endometrial cancer generally shows itself early by abnormal vaginal bleeding. It is treated by hysterectomy

141

(removal of the ovaries, vaginal tract, etc.) prior to spreading of the cancerous cells. Women treated by hysterectomy for endometrial cancer are advised to avoid "hormones" forever, even those patients with history of breast cancer, who face a future of progressive osteoporosis, vaginal atrophy and recurrent urinary tract infections without recourse to hormonal therapy. These women can greatly benefit from natural progesterone therapy.

# Progesterone

Progesterone is the one pro-gestational hormones made by the human body. This is one of the two major female hormone groups (the other is estrogen) made by the ovaries (corpus luteum) starting just prior to ovulation. It is also made in smaller amounts in the adrenal glands in both sexes and the testes in men. After menopause, the adrenal glands are the sole source of progesterone in women.

In pregnant women the placenta, like the corpus luteum, secretes both estrogens and progesterone. The daily production of placental estrogens increases markedly toward the end of pregnancy, by as much as several hundred times the daily production in the middle of a normal monthly cycle.

### *Progesterone effects*

Maintains secretory endometrium

Protects against breast fibrocysts

Helps use fat for energy

Natural diuretic

Natural anti-depressant

Facilitates thyroid hormone action

Normalizes blood clotting

Increases libido

Normalizes blood sugar levels

Restores proper cell oxygen levels

Prevents endometrial cancer and breast cancer

Stimulates osteoblast bone building

Necessary for survival of embryo

Precursor of corticosteroid production

## Progesterone Helps Build Bone

Many postmenopausal women take synthetic estrogen for protection against osteoporosis. Estrogen supplementation has a beneficial effect on osteoclast bone cells for about five years, after which bone loss continues at the same rate as in those women not using estrogen.

Progesterone deficiency causes a decrease in osteoblast-mediated bone formation. Supplemental progesterone has proven to stimulate bone building, while it is not widely prescribed.

## Hormones And Cancer

Both breast and endometrial cancers are health risks that tend to surface in women at a time in their lives when estrogen dominance is likely.

Balance between all circulating hormones and especially the sex hormones, is the key to maintaining good health. An elevated or a depressed level of any one hormone throws off the entire system forcing the body to attempt to compensate for the imbalance.

## Consider the following facts:

❑ Breast cancer is more likely to occur in premenopausal women with normal or high estrogen levels and low progesterone levels. This situation may occur in early adult life in a few women but is quite common after age 35. It also occurs after menopause when women are given estrogen supplements without progesterone.

❑ Among premenopausal women, breast cancer recurrence after mastectomy for breast cancer is more common when surgery has been performed during the first half of the menstrual cycle (when estrogen is dominant) than when surgery had been performed during the latter half (when progesterone is dominant).

❑ Tamoxifen (a weak estrogenic compound that competes with natural estrogen at receptor sites) is commonly prescribed to women after breast cancer surgery for the purpose of preventing recurrence of cancer.

❑ Pregnancy occurring before age 25-30 is known to have a protective effect against breast cancer.

❑ Only the first, full-term, early pregnancy conveys protection. Women having their first pregnancies before age 18 have approximately one-third the risk of women bearing the first child after age 35. Interrupted pregnancies (including spontaneous abortions) do not afford protection and may, in fact, increase the risk of breast cancer.

❑ Women without children are at a higher risk for cancer than those with one or more children.

❑ For women who have had both ovaries removed (oophorectomy) prior to age 30, the risk of breast cancer is significantly reduced.

❑ Protective effects of early oophorectomy is reversed by administration of estrogen.

❑ Treatment of males with estrogen for prostatic cancer or after transsexual surgery is associated with an increased risk of breast cancer.

❑ Industrial pollutants having potent estrogenic effects, called xeno-estrogens, are recognized as a pervasive environmental threat, and a contributing factor in the incidence of breast cancer.

# Dietary Fat And Hormones

A diet high in fat increases serum estrogen, the female sex hormone. Elevated blood serum estrogen is thought to promote breast cancer. However, estrogen isn't significantly lower in vegetarian women on a 30 percent fat intake compared to omnivorous women eating 40 percent of their calories as fat. Reducing dietary fat to 20 percent of total calories would seem to make more sense. Such a reduction did succeed in lowering estrogen levels in premenopausal women. (Boyer)

## Saturated Fat Increases Risk For Sex-Hormone-Related Cancers

International epidemiologic studies show an association between animal fat in the diet and all four of the sex-hormone-related cancers: breast, ovarian and endometrial cancers in women, and prostate cancer in men.

A high correlation exists between the mortality rates from breast and prostate cancer and the amount of dietary animal fat in different countries. Death rates from these cancers are highest in northern Europe and nations with large populations of northern European origin. These people consume the greatest amount of saturated animal fat.

Intermediate mortality rates are found in southern European and Latin American countries, in which an intermediate amount of saturated fat is eaten. The Far East, which has low consumption of animal fat, has the lowest mortality rates for breast and prostate cancers. Dietary fat may be acting directly to influence sex hormone activity, or indirectly, perhaps via prostaglandin and metabolism.

The amount and type of fat in our diet affect our hormones, in particular, the levels of prolactin, estrogen and testosterone. (Hill) Diets high in animal fat encourage the growth of hormone-producing bacteria in the large intestine. Obesity, which is usually the result of a high-fat diet, also affects the hormone levels of the body.

Saturated fat raises blood cholesterol levels. Cholesterol is the precursor to all hormones. Approximately 1,000 milligrams of saturated fat has the same effect on the blood cholesterol level as 25 milligrams of dietary cholesterol. Saturated fat also promotes increased blood clotting which contributes to the development of heart attacks, strokes, gangrene, pulmonary embolism, thromboses, hemorrhoids, and blood clots in the veins of the legs. (Dyerberg, O'Brian)

## In women consuming diets high in animal fats, the following changes are common:

**1.** The onset of maturity in young women occurs early. Girls on healthy,low-fat diets start their menstrual periods at about sixteen years of age. Those on rich diets often begin at age twelve or earlier.

**2.** Menopause occurs approximately four years later on a high fat (50 years versus 46 years).

**3.** Menstrual periods are further apart, longer, heavier, and more painful when fat intake is high.

**4.** Increased levels of these hormones produced may be implemented as a cause of breast cancer.

High-fat diets also cause hormonal changes and early maturation in men, but the effects are not quite as obvious. It may be interesting to speculate about the effects on our society caused by the precocious development of sexual drives and reproductive functions in children.

# Drug and Dietary Influences On Estrogen

## Grapefruit Increases Estrogen Levels

A Swedish study demonstrated that substances found in grapefruit juice, specifically flavonoid glycosides, interact with the metabolism of estrogen and other steroids. After administration of grapefruit juice, peak estrone (between 2-6 hours after tablet intake) concentrations increased significantly in ovariectomized women after a single oral dose intake of 2 mg micronized 17 beta-estradiol. Combined measured estrogens (i.e. estradiol and estrone) also increased significantly.

This study demonstrates that grapefruit juice may alter the metabolic degradation of estrogens, and increase the bioavailable amounts of 17 beta-estradiol and its metabolite estrone, presumably by affecting the oxidative degradation of estrogens. This food interaction may be one factor behind the individual variabilities in 17 beta-estradiol, estrone and estriol serum concentrations after administration of 17 beta-estradiol to patients. (Schubert)

## Ascorbic Acid and Acetaminophen Increase Estrogen

Concentrations of estrogen may be increased by ascorbic acid (vitamin C) and acetaminophen which compete with it in the gut wall. Theoretically, problems may arise if these agents are stopped suddenly. (Shenfield)

## Antihistamines Decrease Estrogen, but not Progesterone

Seldane™ (generic name: terfenadine), an over the counter antihistamine marketed to reduce symptoms of allergies, has shown to decrease estrogen and progesterone levels. Histamine has a direct stimulatory effect on steroid production in the body.

In a trial at the University Women's Hospital of Tubingen, Germany, progesterone and estradiol production were measured in the presence and absence of histamine and terfenadine. Histamine stimulated a dose-related increase in estradiol secretion. This response was blocked specifically by the antihistamine terfenadine. Progesterone production in response to histamine stimulation was independent of dose. This effect may have a physiological role in the menstrual cycle. (Bodis)

This information infers that antihistamine medications such as Seldane™ may reduce the effectiveness of birth control pills, or interfere with hormone balances, possibly contributing to menstrual related disturbances.

## Antibiotics Decrease Effectiveness of Birth Control

Effectiveness of oral contraceptives may be influenced by various drugs. The *Archives of Dermatology* (March 1994) printed a letter titled *"Frequency of pregnancy in acne patients taking oral antibiotics and oral contraceptives."* (London) This letter reveals the magnitude of the associated problems.

Impaired effectiveness of oral contraceptives results in breakthrough bleeding or pregnancy. Effectiveness may be reduced due to impairment of their enterohepatic circulation. This may be due to absorption of estrogen conjugates or to insufficient intestinal bacteria. Broad spectrum antibiotics such as ampicillin and neomycin indiscriminately destroy bacteria throughout the body, not just the bacteria causing the infection or problem. (Bolt) Without healthy normally present intestinal bacterial, digestion and absorption are less than optimal.

Normally, estrogens (but not progesterone) are metabolized in the liver and then recirculated. Antibiotics may interfere with this process reducing plasma levels of active estrogen hormones. It is not certain if this is true for all women or for a subgroup of women.

Antifungal agents can also inhibit estrogen metabolism and increase its plasma concentrations.

Oral contraceptives can also interfere with the metabolism or activity of other therapeutic agents. Oral contraceptives may induce metabolism of other drugs which are glucuronidated, including some benzodiazepines (such as Valium™) and analgesics. The clinical significance of this type of interaction is also unknown. (Shenfield)

# A Word About Birth Control Pills

Contraceptives which contain a combination of varying amounts of synthetic estrogen and progesterone, inhibit the production of natural hormones. They work by inhibiting the normal interaction of sex hormones and the pituitary gland. Use of birth control pills causes more than unnatural hormone regulation:

**1.** Contraceptives elevate triglycerides, often to abnormal levels. Contraceptives, taken regularly, also increase your chances of stroke or heart attack, because they raise all of the other lipids almost as much as 30 percent or more. The pill is a proven and accepted causative agent in cerebrovascular and heart disease. It

149

increases risk of some forms of cancer, causes a wide array of nutritional problems, and is strongly suspected as a cause of diabetes.

**2.** Some combinations of progesterone and estrogen are worse than others. Norethitdrone ethynodiol diacetate and nestrarol elevate triglycerides. Estrogens raise phospholipids and triglycerides and lower cholesterol. (*Fertility and Sterility*) If you have high cholesterol or other elevated lipid, you should beware of contraceptive use. If your blood pressure is already over the normal limit, birth control medication may raise it even higher.

**3.** Women using birth control pills experience more vaginitis. It is believed that contraceptive pills prevent the production of normal hormone generated mucus which would prevent infection. (Lee) (DHEA increases this mucus.)

### *If the pill is so dangerous, why do so many women still take it?*

Unfortunately, for the most part, the ill effects of birth control pills, (and most other synthetic hormone analogs and many drugs) are down played by the medical and pharmaceutical communities. It is convenient and many are just plain uninformed. Doctors don't warn women of the possibilities of vaginitis, blood clots, stroke, or even death.

## Natural Hormone Replacement Therapy and DHEA

Menopause is associated with a reduction in DHEA levels. In one study, the average plasma level of DHEA was 542 in premenopausal women, 197 in postmenopausal women, and only 126 in a woman whose ovaries had been surgically removed.

(Monroe) In a group of women between the ages of 55 and 85 years, there was a significant correlation between serum levels of DHEA-S and bone density of the vertebral spine. (Wild) Women with higher levels of DHEA had greater bone mass than those with lower DHEA levels.

In young females, the ovaries are responsible for 50 percent of androgen production and the remainder coming from conversion of DHEA. With aging, the ovary, despite estrogen loss, is still able to synthesize androgens. However, clinical estrogen substitution does nothing to restore DHEA levels, suggesting a non-estrogen dependent role for ovarian function in regulating DHEA production. (Cumming) Removal of the ovaries has shown to have a significant influence on DHEA levels enhancing the age related decline. However, DHEA decline is probably indicative of changes in the adrenals. The implications of this suggests that the other androgens whose levels are fairly stable despite aging may have more psychological importance to the maintenance of youthful survival which may go beyond their role as sex steroids.

# Postmenopausal Hormone Replacement

A recent study in postmenopausal women concluded that DHEA benefits estrogen therapy. DHEA protects against neoplasia, osteoporosis, and cardiac disease, and DHEA should be effective in treating the decline in function due to menopause. (Buster)

Supplemental DHEA given orally has proven to be highly beneficial. Healthy women given DHEA rapidly convert it to estrogens causing a 300-500 percent temporary increase in levels. Testosterone levels also temporarily increase by 300-400 percent. These effects occur only if the body naturally requires such a conversion. Therefore, supplemental DHEA is non-toxic and far safer than taking synthetic hormones or steroids.

Dr. Joel Hargrove studied the safety and efficacy of "natural" estradiol (E2) and progesterone in menopause women with moderate to severe symptoms compared to women on synthetic analogs. He found the following results:

❑ Estrogens rose significantly from baseline in both groups.

❑ Progesterone increased significantly above baseline in the natural group, but did not change in the synthetic group.

❑ All women on E2 and progesterone had a decrease in total cholesterol and an increase in HDL cholesterol.

❑ Those on synthetic conjugated estrogens and progesterone acetate had no significant change from baseline in total cholesterol; however, they did have an increase in HDL (high-density lipoprotein) cholesterol.

❑ After six months, in the E2 and progesterone group, there was no uterine bleeding. Four of five women on the synthetics continued regular withdrawal bleeding throughout the study period, but they experienced no endometrial cell development.

This study demonstrates that the daily administration of a combination of micronized E2 and progesterone results in symptomatic improvement, minimal side effects, an improved lipid profile, and amenorrhea without endometrial abnormal cell proliferation in menopause women. (Hargrove)

# DHEA and Pregnancy

During pregnancy, DHEA is derived from both fetal and maternal metabolism. During the last weeks of pregnancy, the maternal DHEA decreases by one third while fetal adrenal DHEA production increases. Fetal membranes or placenta may play a role in DHEA metabolism. DHEA tests have been used in an attempt to delineate fetal growth retardation. A decrease in DHEA in the placenta of women with severe pre-eclampsia may explain the decline in plasma and urinary estrogen levels in women with this problem. The level of DHEA is elevated in women with cervical ripening preceding the onset of labor.

# DHEA and Hair Growth

The role of DHEA in hair growth has been associated with hirsutism or hair loss in women. A correlation between DHEA levels and male pattern baldness exists in young men.

Hair contains high quantities of DHEA. High concentrations of DHEA or testosterone sulfate found in hair is a function of adjacent sweat glands while free steroids found are derived from sebaceous glands. DHEA and AED may be key factors in preventing hair loss caused by G-6-PD enzyme. (Kasick)

In patients with hirsutism, suppression of ACTH production with dexamethasone results in decreases in androgen / DHEA production with slowing of hair growth. In contrast, with treatment to decrease serum testosterone concentration but not DHEA, there is still a decline in hair growth. DHEA stimulated hair growth in mice and guinea pigs although it did block induced growth of vibrissae on prolonged administration. (Shapiro)

The skin contains the enzymes necessary to convert DHEA to dihydrotestosterone or testosterone. In support of this, higher levels are found in acne patients. There is a correlation between DHEA and androgen levels with acne and hair density in men. There is also a relationship between male pattern baldness and DHEA levels.

# Chapter Summary

This complicated chapter reviews the complex relationship between DHEA and the male and female reproductive systems. While DHEA has been reported by many individuals to increase libido, clinical trials have not yet conclusively proven this. DHEA is discussed in relationship to male and female reproductive capabilities, and other hormone related situations such as prostate cancer and menopause. Menopause is associated with a reduction in DHEA levels. DHEA is discussed as a possible safer alternative to hormone replacement therapy.

# WILD YAM: NATURAL PROGESTERONE

The medicinal properties of wild yams, not to be confused with the sweet potato, have actually been known for a long time by folk herbalists prior to pharmaceutical manufacturers. Daniel Mowrey reported in *The Scientific Validation of Herbal Medicine* that throughout the 18th and 19th centuries wild yam was used to treat menstrual cramps and problems related to childbirth. As far back as 25 B.C. the Mexican wild yam was mentioned in the Pen Tsao Ching by the Chinese who highly valued the herb.

Mexican wild yam was a primary source of the production of synthetic progesterone and other hormones for a number of years. Until recently, wild yam was the sole source of the diosgenin used in making contraceptive pills.

According to herbalist Rosemary Gladstar in *Herbal Healing for Women*, wild yam is "the most widely used herb in the world today." Over 200 million prescriptions that contain its derivatives are sold each year. Diosgenin continues to provide about 50 percent of the raw material for steroid synthesis and is a multi-billion dollar industry.

# Hormone History

Cholesterol is the precursor of all hormones in the body. Cholesterol was first isolated in the 1700's, but the first investigator to become interested in the nature of cholesterol was Windhaus, a German scientist, now considered "the father of sterol chemistry." Windhaus had a brilliant student, Adolph Butenandt, who was directed by Windhaus to investigate the hormone substance from the urine of pregnant women which induced heat in mice and rats. This research resulted in the isolation and identification of the estrogen called estrone.

While Butenandt had extracted testosterone from animal sources he wanted to synthesize this substance. He instead was able to synthesize a precursor to testosterone, DHEA. The first extractions were from cholesterol, the ultimate hormone precursor. With the second extraction method, he was able to extract DHEA from beta sitosterol, a plant sterol available from many different oils such as soy.

In the late 1920's, the University of Chicago Professor of Physiologic Chemistry, Fred C. Koch, and his student, Lemuel McGee, were on the trail of the male hormone from extracts from bull testes. Teaming up with an Irish researcher, Dr. T. F. Gallagher, they utilized an extraction process that yielded an improved mixture.

Testosterone was immediately recognized by physicians as a sex hormone that had muscle building properties, etc. For years body builders, weight lifters, and athletes have used anabolic steroids to gain strength, weight, and muscle mass. The side effects, cancer, leukemia, kidney disease, sterility, violent mood swings, make this a dangerous practice.

# Wild Mexican Yam as Source of Progesterone

In 1936 Japanese researchers realized that an extract of the yam, termed diosgenin, was remarkably similar to some of the adrenal hormones and to the precursor molecule, cholesterol.

In 1943, Professor Russell Marker of the University of Pennsylvania discovered a rich hormone source in the wild, the Barbasco yam. He developed a method for economically extracting hormones and assigned the patents to Parke Davis. He discovered they had no registered patents in Mexico so he proceeded to set up his own extraction facility.

He travelled to Mexico and became intrigued with the Shamans, the "medicine men." He was familiar with hormonal chemistry and that certain plant substances were used by "medicine men" throughout Central and South America and China. He knew that certain yams were being used for birth control and to treat female problems, so he theorized that there were some hormonal properties present in the  specific species of wild yam, the Barbasco Yam.

Barbasco Yams have black tubers which grow under the ground with vines growing on top. These yams were wildcrafted in mountainous regions. He spoke with locals to learn exactly how they prepared and used the yams.

Marker presented a bag of a powdered white substance to one of the Mexican Pharmaceutical companies involved in hormone research and processing, Hormoneasa. He claimed the bag contained progesterone which he derived from the Barbasco yam, and asked for $800.00. This was hard for them to believe as at that time progesterone and estrogen were derived only through expensive chemical extraction methods from animal urine at a cost of approximately $3,000 a kilo. They tested Marker's product and found it to be pure progesterone. Needless to say, they were amazed. They immediately contacted him to persuade him to sell his technology but were unsuccessful. He had no intentions

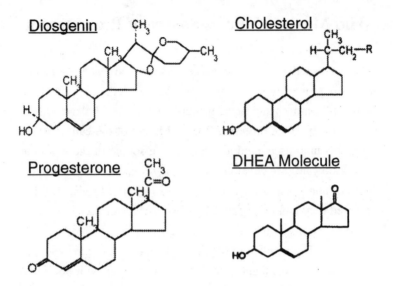

*Note that Diosgenin is closer in structure to progesterone than it is to DHEA.*

of divulging his secrets.

Several American pharmaceutical companies travelled to Mexico to try to buy his technology but were also unsuccessful. Marker opted to produce it himself and supply them with the raw material. Numerous pharmaceutical companies sent in their own biochemists to try to follow him and trick him into revealing his method.

He eventually left Mexico and never sold out. In time others were able to develop their own means of synthesizing progesterone. This is what began the "hormone frenzy" across the world, giving the Barbasco Yam its great value.

The raw material is loaded with precursor phytogenins, including diosgenin, which today is easily enzymatically used to manufacture DHEA progesterone and many other hormones. Diosgenin is remarkably similar to progesterone and is believed to be used in the body as progesterone. Diosgenin may also be used as a progesterone intermediate.

While other sources of plant steroids are available for

158

such purposes - such as soybeans, agave and yucca - wild yam is the best, most concentrated source.

# Value of Yams Increases Dramatically

Following Marker's discovery these yams created a booming steroid industry in Mexico. In 1951 *Fortune Magazine* ran an article that claimed the steroid industry created "the biggest technological boom ever heard south of the border." Over the next 20 to 30 years the value of these yams increased dramatically as just a few companies through political ties with the Mexican government, were completely monopolizing this technology by controlling the growing and harvesting of the Barbasco Yam. The yams were shipped to Europe to be processed into pharmaceutical hormones.

The steroid hormone business exploded during this time as the yams provided an easier, much less expensive, way to manufacture hormones. Birth control pills and all sorts of hormone therapies for menopausal women and for those who have undergone hysterectomies were introduced at this time.

Many companies were after this technology and tried to buy it, steal it, or somehow duplicate it within their own laboratories. Numerous original patents came out at this time. Manufacturing firms started manipulating molecules in order to apply for their own patents.

Patents protect products from competitors from duplicating it, undercutting the price, and stealing the originator's profits. A great deal of time, testing, and money goes into product development. It is not ethical for a competitor to produce the same thing, and reap the profits from another's work. A patent is like directions for the development of a product which is unique to the manufacturer.

Companies can obtain patents for a product in such a

way so as not to disclose all privileged information about making that product. This prevents competitors from having enough information to steal their product, as there was a great deal of this going on.

Approximately 200 million prescriptions are written every year for yam-based products, specifically synthetic hormones which are derived from the yams. This presents a multi-billion dollar industry within this area of pharmaceutical hormones alone.

# Yams and Progesterone

Diosgenin, extracted from Mexican wild yams, and human steroids, are not the same. If a yam extract has steroidal effects on the body, it is not because it actually contains steroidal hormones, but because the steroidal-like precursors have similar effects. The body does not recognize precursors or mistake them for its own natural hormones, but uses them in a similar manner.

The *British Herbal Pharmacopoeia* recognizes wild yam root as a spasmolytic, mild diaphoretic, anti-inflammatory, anti-rheumatic and cholagogue, and for use in the treatment of: Intestinal Colic, Diverticulitis, Rheumatoid Arthritis, Muscular Rheumatism, Cramps, Intermittent Claudification (leg clots), Cholecystitis, Dysmenorrhea, Ovarian and Uterine Pain.

Although many physicians believe that there is no significant difference between synthetic and natural progesterones, others disagree, such as New York City obstetrician, Dr. Neils Lauerson, M.D., author of *PMS: Premenstrual Syndrome and You.* Lauerson says that some synthetic progesterones can have masculinizing effects on a woman while others cause fluid retention. Natural progesterone from wild yam, on the other hand, does not cause masculinization, and is known to reduce sodium and fluid retention.

John Lee, M.D., of Sebastopol, California, says that the reason synthetic progesterone causes side effects is because, "It is not progesterone. Pharmaceutical companies alter the molecular structure so it (referring to synthetic progesterone analogs) no longer fits into the biochemical machinery of the body."

The progesterone taken from the wild yam, on the other hand, is nearly identical to what the body produces, Lee explains. And the body easily converts it into the identical molecule it needs. That is not the case with synthetic compounds, and this is the main reason for side effects associated with synthetic hormones.

## Yams: Anti-inflammatory /Anti-arthritic

Animal and human studies have demonstrated diosgenin to have beneficial effects on cholesterol and hypertension. Dioscorea induced a short-lived decrease in blood pressure and an increase in coronary flow when injected intravenously into rabbits. Also in rabbits, the saponins of yams, fed orally, prevented large increases in blood cholesterol levels. The beneficial therapeutic effect of dioscorea saponins on patients with atherosclerosis combined with hypertension was confirmed in clinical practice. (Lewis)

Yams have long been used to make cortisone, a very common anti-inflammatory agent used for everything from rashes to joint inflammation.

## Yams and Osteoporosis

Clinical studies have shown that all postmenopausal women, aged 38 to 83, using a cream with natural hormone compounds extracted from wild yams, increased bone density levels.

Some women increased their bone density levels as much as 25 percent. Unlike synthetic estrogen, these compounds actually restore bone density. The various hormonal effects of DHEA appear to decrease bone reabsorption and increase bone formation. There have been no noted side effects with natural wild yam cream. (Lee)

# Natural vs. Synthetic Progesterone

The effects of natural and synthetic hormones differ greatly. Synthetic progestins do not match the body's chemistry and can inhibit ovulation and suppress the body's production of its own natural progesterone. Progestins are used in oral contraceptives and in Provera™, commonly prescribed to menopausal women. If a doctor thinks a woman has a hormonal imbalance, he or she may prescribe synthetic progestins — which may aggravate the symptoms rather than eliminate them. Many women become irritable, ill-tempered and emotionally unstable on Provera™.

In spite of the known side effects and risks, doctors today prescribe synthetic progesterone for women with menstrual problems, osteoporosis, and menopausal symptoms.

Some doctors say they don't wish to prescribe natural progesterone because it is not FDA approved for PMS. Progesterone is an approved drug for other uses. The FDA does not approve or disapprove of how a drug is used by a doctor. Such "unapproved" uses may be appropriate and may reflect approaches to drug therapy that have been extensively reported in medical literature. Provera™ is frequently prescribed for the treatment of menopause. However, the FDA has never "approved" Provera™ for menopause either.

Many women may feel remarkably better by substituting natural progesterone for Provera™. Progesterone usually improves PMS. New studies show that natural progesterone may be more important than estrogen in the prevention of osteoporosis. A cream containing natural progesterone from wild yam is safer than conventional pharmaceuticals.

## Natural vs. Synthetic Estrogens

The issue of natural versus synthetic hormones is also important to women taking estrogen. A study in Sweden showed an increase in breast cancer among women using high doses of synthetic estrogen called ethinyl estradiol - a substance used in lower doses in oral contraceptives in the U.S. By contrast, the doses of natural estrogen used postmenopausally are about 10 to 20 times lower than the synthetic estrogen in the pill. Physicians often put adolescent girls on birth control pills with high levels of synthetic estrogens, but are reluctant to give women with premenopausal symptoms the low doses of natural estrogens they need.

Premarin™ and Provera™ are the most widely prescribed combination drugs for hormone replacement therapy in menopausal women, but many women experience problems with Premarin™. Premarin™ is estrogen made from the urine of pregnant horses, and while it is natural for horses, it is not necessarily for humans, and can cause numerous side-effects.

*Note:* There is much controversy over the way that this drug is manufactured. According to the animal activist group, Friends of Animals, to collect the key ingredient for Premarin™, mares are kept pregnant nearly their entire lives and are confined to stalls so small that they are unable to turn around during seven of their 11 months of pregnancy. Once born their newborns are slaughtered, as "unwanted by-products of the manufacturing process." This slaughtering claimed over 75,000 horses in 1993.

Synthetic estrogens, including conjugated equine

(horse) estrogens, ethinyl estradiol, and diethylstilbestrol, are very stressful to the kidneys. Synthetic progestins have variable effects on lipoproteins. In particular, the 19 nor-testosterone derivatives including norgestrel norethindrone, norethindrone acetate, and norethisterone, increase concentrations of LDL cholesterol - the "bad" cholesterol - and reduce HDL - the "good" cholesterol. This potentially reduces the beneficial cardiovascular effects of estrogen.

Synthetic progestins also exert a detrimental but less significant effect on these lipoproteins, but also reduce sex hormone-binding globulin, resulting in an increase in free sex hormone levels and potentially increased androgenicity.

Natural progesterone preparations, like those from the wild yam, administered orally can produce excellent blood levels without unwanted effects such as fluid retention, breast tenderness, weight gain, and depression caused by the synthetics. Correspondingly, oral natural E2 and progesterone would seem preferable for long-term replacement therapy. (Hargrove)

## Chapter Summary

Wild Mexican yams contain Diosgenin, which is chemically similar to cholesterol and progesterone. Diosgenin is the raw material used to manufacture progesterone, cortisone and many other steroid hormones today. Diosgenin has therapeutic properties of its own but because of its similarity to DHEA and progesterone, in the body, it is believed to act as, to mimic, or to precurse progesterone.

Synthetic hormones are known to have numerous and dangerous side effects. It is far better to produce these hormones naturally, eliminating these dangers. Diosgenin is found in many oral or topical products as the molecules are small enough to be absorbed into the skin transdermally.

# TESTIMONIALS

*"Words nor paper can describe what this wild yam cream has done for me! Within 4 days my flashes had decreased to at least 1/3 and were only 1/3 as bad. After using the first jar (2 1/2) weeks my hot flashes are almost completely gone. I truly feel this cream was made just for me."* C.C.

*"I feel like dancing again! I feel that wonderful, thanks to this wild yam cream. Thank-you, Thank-you!"* G.C.

*"My menstrual periods were very, very irregular. I was amazed when I got a period after taking wild yam cream for only 7 days. My hot flashes have stopped and I feel great."* C.P.

*"Thank-you for introducing this wild yam cream into the market. It has saved my outlook on life."* Y.D.

*"I dreaded the thought of approaching my "change of life," but with your product, the transition has been a gentle, almost satisfying experience."* H.R.

*"For years I have suffered with PMS and feelings of discomfort every month. Since I started using your wild yam cream, I noticed a major difference in the very first month. Thank-you."* L.L.

*"I could actually feel a difference the first time I applied the wild yam cream. I have tried hormone replacement therapy and found the side effects to be too harsh. Thanks!"* I.H.

*"I felt an increased amount of energy using the wild yam extract - I was able to handle stressful situations much easier"* A.M.

*"I have lost 15 pounds since I starting taking wild yam extract. I haven't felt•like this for over 20 years. At 63 years old I am starting to live again. I find myself stronger, more energetic and active.... Also, I desire sex once again."* C.C.

*"The wild yam extract has definitely made a difference in my workout. I feel stronger and more energetic. I receive comments from people all the time in regards to my great strength. Many people think I am taking steroids, but it's completely natural and without the danger and without the side effects."* K.J.

*"After taking wild yam for 6 months, my memory problem has improved by 90-95%. My sex drive has improved 200-300%. My general feelings, awareness, is better today than it has been in 10 years or more. Everyone should know about DHEA and wild yam."* F.R.

*"I tried the wild yam and felt that stress was much easier to deal with. I felt stronger in the gym and lost some body fat. A lot of people commented upon how good I looked."* B.N.

# DHEA TESTIMONIALS:

*"I have been taking DHEA sublingually for 3 years and have lost over 20 lbs. It's great stuff!"* J.S.D.

*"Since using DHEA my lean body mass has definitely increased and it's easier to keep the belly fat off."* J.M.

*"This DHEA stuff is so powerful I can only take 25 mg every other day! I am loaded with energy, but I sleep great at night. It's pretty amazing."* J.J.

*"People think I am about 20 years younger than I am all the time. I just say thank-you, but really I think it's the DHEA."* M.P.

*"I was taking DHEA for years before it became available over the counter. It's incredible what sacrifices the public has had to put up with because of this countries stubborn bureaucratic system. Everyone should have the legal right to something that can do so much good for our health. I wouldn't be without it no matter what the law says."* BH

*"I used to have to wait to get this stuff (DHEA) from Europe. It's a lot more convenient now. Soon it will be in every health food store and pharmacy. I have lost weight and know I am much healthier in general. Thanks for the great book. It's about time people found out about DHEA."* no name

*"My wife has suffered from colitis from some time. Her doctors used to prescribe cortisone all the time. With DHEA she has a lot more energy, feels better and without any side effects."* N.A.

*"I just started taking DHEA and was surprised to find that it really worked. I feel great, sleep great, don't have to work so hard to keep my weight down. I want more!"* M.P.

*"I give it (DHEA) to both my parents who suffer from arthritis. They think I have given them the miracle cure of the next century."* B.C.

*"I have asthma and sometimes have sinus problems. I found that opening a capsule and placing the DHEA under my tongue or using one or two drops of the liquid sublingual brings me instant relief!"* B.M.

*"I have been using DHEA for the last several months and have a tremendous energy increase, but people need to be aware of its potential side effects. This is a great book- the best I have found on this subject. Thank-you!"* C.M.

*"I have arthritis in my ankles and knees. It is very painful, especially in the morning. DHEA Sublingual gives me almost instant relief so that I can get up and do what I need to do, It really works!"* W.P.

*"I have Lupus and have been so sick that for long periods I didn't get out of bed. Since I have been using DHEA, and especially the sublingual, my life has changed. I carry the sublingual with me wherever I go because if I need it, it works so fast! I don't have any side effects even if I take 200 mg encapsuled a day."* J.M.

*"I have noticed that DHEA really helps keep the body fat off. I feel better and leaner!"* N.J.

*"I can testify that DHEA definitely boosts your sex drive!"* G.W.

*"I have lost 30 pounds and my shin looks at least 10 years younger since I have been using SkinGuard\* with DHEA and Pregnenolone. It gives me incredible energy."* C.B.

*"I have noticed a definite reduction in size and lightening of color of age spots on my hands since I starting using SkinGuard\* cream."* D.D.

\* SkinGuard, manufactured by VitalSource, AMEC, Inc. (714-452-0427), is a cream containing DHEA and Pregnenolone utilizing a transdermal liposome delivery system.

# HOW TO USE DHEA RESPONSIBLY

The availability of free form DHEA over the counter in the United States has brought us (consumers) into an entirely new area of "self-care" and responsibility. If we expect the government to continue to allow availability of such powerful substances than we must realize that the manner in which we choose to utilize them may determine the length of their availability.

To many Americans seem to hold onto the idea that if a little is good, then more is better. In actuality, the opposite is true. For this reason, the regulatory agencies have had to take action and "control" certain substances such as pain killers. Taking too much may have serious detrimental and often addictive effects. Pharmacists monitor frequency of refills, and "triplicate" prescriptions prevent individuals from getting these medications filled at more than one pharmacy.

I shook my head when I saw 200 and 300 mg capsules available to the public. This is way too high for DHEA to be used as an "anti-aging" dose and too high for use without the supervision of a doctor.

I shuddered when I heard about individuals taking mega doses as high as 1,600 mg. daily to lose weight. Just because one study showed that this amount taken for 30 days produced a dramatic reduction in body fat, does not by any means indicate that this is a safe and recommended dosage for the public, and especially for longer than 30 days and without a doctors supervision. These are some of the reasons I felt so strongly compelled to inform supplemental DHEA users of th facts and urge caution.

The potential negative effects of supplemental DHEA on the liver are very disturbing to me. I realize that many people do utilize antioxidants, many people do not and many people should probably be taking higher amounts than they do. Lastly, I have been recently introduced to a fascinating little-known antioxidant that when taken with DHEA actually can prevent the stress on the liver from the DHEA.

Before we can go any further in our discussion on using DHEA responsibly, we must review the different delivery systems.

# DHEA DELIVERY SYSTEMS

Physicians around the world, including Dr. Richard Ash of the Ash Comprehensive Medicine Clinic in New York, have determined that delivery systems are of critical importance in obtaining the optimal results for their patients using DHEA and Pregnenolone.

## Capsules and Tablets

Although this is the most popular way to take DHEA, it is the worst. Side effects are most likely to occur with this delivery system and assimilation is the lowest - only 30 to 50 percent of what is in the capsules or tablet actually enters the blood stream.

Capsules and tablets also pose a possible stress to the liver as it must be swallowed and must pass through the liver before reaching the blood stream.

Animal studies using incredibly high dosages of

DHEA demonstrated possible liver stress and increased cancer risk, however, if a 100 lb. humans were to take the amounts that the rats did (.45 percent of their total body weight) they would have to take approximately 90 bottles of 25 mg capsules per day.

The breakdown of testosterone and estrogens is very high among capsules and tablets, increasing the risk of side effects.

## Transdermals

Creams and patches are also a popular way to supplement DHEA and Pregnenolone, but it is not the best. Assimilation is higher, 50 to 85 percent depending on the quality of the cream, what carriers are present, thickness of the skin (thinner creams have higher absorption compared to thicker creams), where the cream is applied (thin skin or fatty areas), cleanliness of skin and humidity.

A major disadvantage of transdermals is the fact that the hormones remain in the fat cells under the skin where they are stored and released very slowly. Toxic levels can build up rapidly and remain so for prolonged periods even after one stops using the cream.

To help ward off potential problems with hormone storage with transdermals, do not use more than the recommended dosage on the product or by your physician. Be sure to cycle your dosages by using the cream for three weeks, then stop for at least a week. Have your hormone levels checked frequently to determine how much you are storing in your body. You may find that after using the cream for a few months that you need to stop using it for longer than one week

A unique advantage of transdermals is that they can be applied directly to melanomas or age spots and doctors are seeing positive effects. Melanomas **are actually reducing**

171

and age spots are lightening.

Transdermal delivery of DHEA eliminates the liver first pass, and therefore is safer for the liver.

### Liquid Sublinguals and Liposome Sprays

This is the best way to supplement DHEA or Pregnenolone. There is fast, direct assimilation into the blood stream through the thin mucousal membranes of the mouth, avoiding the liver first pass. The assimilation is much higher 95 to 100 percent. Used properly, there are fewer side effects as there is less conversion to other hormones such as testosterone and estrogen which can cause problems in women.

# DHEA Dosages

Although DHEA is a steroid it does not seem to exhibit the strong hormone influences of "fully formed" steroids like estrogen, testosterone, or progesterone. As a consequence, this steroid "precursor" possess a minimal anabolic, androgenic and estrogenic activity.

Ideal supplemental DHEA dosage can vary dramatically from person to person. Age is a strong factor, but other biological influences may be significant, including your ability to absorb and assimilate the supplement. Our ability to absorb and assimilate decrease as we grow older. Some people recommend do that DHEA be taken on an empty stomach to improve assimilation, while this is not always necessary for all people. Normal DHEA dosages range from 5-50 mg., taking into consideration what delivery system you are using. If you have *any* question as to what your individual proper dosage is, before and after tests of blood or saliva DHEA levels are recommended to assess your proper dose.

Anti-aging doses would be quite low, taking only enough to raise your levels to a normal 20 year old, (approximately 31 mg. in men, 19 mg. in women). Because men naturally manufacture higher amounts than women do, men can take higher supplemental amounts.

## Safe, long-term preventative "anti-aging" DHEA daily supplementation:

| | Women | Men |
|---|---|---|
| **Capsules or Tablets** | 5 to 25 mg. | 5 to 50 mg. |
| **Transdermals** | 5 to 15 mg. | 5 to 25 mg. |
| **Sublinguals or Sprays** | 5 to 10 mg. | 5 to 25 mg. |

Therapeutic doses may be much higher than 50 mg, encapsulated daily. New studies show us that capsules may not be the ideal delivery system for those using DHEA therapeutically because of the additional stress to the liver.

Many physicians prescribing over 50 mg. encapsulated dosages daily recommend cycling, taking DHEA daily for 4 weeks, then taking 2 to 4 weeks off, before starting the next cycle. This is to protect the adrenal glands, liver and promote continued optimal production. Cycling is not necessary if using sublingual or spray delivery systems.

As with other steroid hormones, it is recommended that intake levels begin low and gradually increase to the proper dose. It is also suggested that if you wish to stop taking DHEA, one should not suddenly stop, but slowly decrease the dosage to "wean" yourself off.

If you do experience side effects, such as acne or unwanted hair growth, and in some cases, irritability and rapid heart beat, the amount you are taking may be too high and you should reduce the dosage.

# Test Yourself

Getting your hormone levels tested before you begin taking DHEA, Pregnenolone or any other hormone is the only responsible way. You then need to do a follow up test to ensure that you are in the desirable range. With saliva test kits now readily available, this is simple and inexpensive to do. You can determine first of all whether you are a candidate for supplementation. Many individuals under the age of 40 are anxious to start supplementing DHEA without realizing that it could be detrimental if it is not warranted. Granted, many health problems may cause one's DHEA level to drop faster than a "healthy" individual, but one can not be certain without having a sample analyzed.

### Saliva Tests: Just as Accurate as Blood Tests

Testing saliva instead of blood offers a convenient and reliable methods of determining your hormonal status. Blood tests for a single hormone can range from $90 to $150. A saliva test at this writing is $40 to $45.

Saliva tests measure "free" hormones - the biologically active form. Only 3 to 5 percent of a specific hormone is free and capable of producing effects on tissues. The remaining 95 percent or more is bound - tied to sex steroid-binding globulins - and the bound molecule is too large to pass into the saliva.

## Normal Female A.M. DHEA Levels in Saliva

| AGE | RANGE |
|-----|-------|
| 20-29 | 129-177 pg/ml |
| 30-39 | 75-185 |
| 40-49 | 97-123 |
| 50-59 | 85-115 |
| 60-69 | 49-61 |
| 70-79 | 35-41 |

## Normal Male A.M. DHEA Levels in Saliva

| AGE | RANGE |
|-----|-------|
| 20-29 | 280-288 pg/ml |
| 30-39 | 172-248 |
| 40-49 | 94-128 |
| 50-59 | 85-111 |
| 60-69 | 61-83 |
| 70-79 | 54-86 |

To avoid side effects and long term complications one would not want to be above 288 pg/ml for males and 177 pg/ml for females.

**The following are diagnostic laboratories offering salivary hormonal assay tests:**

> Aeron Lifecycles          800-631-7900
> 1933 Davis Street, suite 310
> San Leandro, CA 94577

> Diagnos-Techs, Inc.          800-878-3787
> Clinical and Research Laboratory
> 6620 South 192nd Pl. J-104
> Kent, WA  98032

> Great Smokies Diagnostic Laboratory   704-253-0621
> 18 A. Regent Park Blvd.
> Asheville, NC 28806
> 704-253-0621

> National Biotech Laboratory          800-846-6285
> 13758 Lake City Way, N.E.
> Seattle, WA 98125

When ordering a saliva test kit you will usually prepay for the desired number of tests desired. You will receive sample collection materials, instructions and a mailer to use to send the sample to the laboratory. Results are returned to you within five to seven working days.

# DHEA: SIDE EFFECTS

DHEA has wide past clinical experience and is remarkably free of side effects **WHEN TAKEN IN THE PROPER AMOUNT**, especially when compared to conventional treatments.

DHEA when taken in amounts greater than what the body needs can produce undesirable effects. In excess, DHEA becomes a stress on the body instead of a stress reducer.

Signals that your supplemental DHEA intake may be **TOO HIGH** include the following:

> **Acne**
>
> **Facial hair (women)**
>
> **Rapid heart beat**
>
> **Irritability/ Anxiety**
>
> **Headaches**
>
> **Sleep disruption**

If you experience any of these while taking DHEA you should **REDUCE YOUR INTAKE**. For optimal results, contact a healthcare practitioner familiar with DHEA who can monitor your levels through blood or saliva tests.

**Contraindications for DHEA use:**

> Pregnant women
>
> Individuals under age 25
>
> Women with a history of breast cancer
>
> Men with pre-existing prostate cancer

Women prone to development of ovarian cysts should avoid capsules, but may consider sublingual or spray delivery systems if low DHEA levels are present.

# DHEA Effects on the Liver

A research team lead by Leon Milewich at The University of Texas, Southwestern Medical Center in Dallas, Texas, presented data pertaining to some of the in vivo effects associated with dietary DHEA administration to mice and rats. A number of studies have reported that dietary DHEA leads to the following liver changes: (Wu)

**(1) Decrease in total body weight gain; but with relative increases in liver weight;**

**(2) Liver color change;** DHEA supplementation results in the change of liver color from a normal pink to mahogany, peroxisome proliferation in liver cells and alterations in liver cell mitochondria.

**(3) Apparent increases in the levels of 26 proteins and decreases in the levels of 7 proteins** including phosphorylation and carbamoyl phosphate synthetase-I(CPS-I),

**(4) Increased liver enzymes** (peroxisomal enzymes; I,AMPase and OTPase; cytosolic malic enzymes; glutathione 5-transferase) A protein identified as carbamoyl phosphate synthetase-I(CPS-I), was decreased markedly by DHEA action. This enzyme,which comprises approximately 15-20 percent of mitochondrial matrix protein,is involved in the entry and rate-limiting step of the urea cycle. The specific activity of CPS-I also was significantly decreased by DHEA, but serum urea levels were normal.

**(5)** Decreased hepatic mitochondrial cross-sectional area.

**(6) Significant decreases** in the hepatic rates of **fatty acid** and **cholesterol synthesis.**

**(7)** formation of 5-androstene-3p,17p-diol as a major metabolite of DHEA by subcellular fractions of liver, which is reflected in serum and tissue levels.

University of Texas Southwestern Medical Center at Dallas reported that DHEA administration resulted in profound changes in the sodium dodecylsulfate-polyacrylamide gel electrophoresis patterns of endogenous radiophosphorylated proteins. (Cecil)

### If you were a rat...

In animal studies the supplemental DHEA dosage given daily is usually around .45 percent of their total body weight. (As noted in the study you enclosed.) Sometimes, (not surprisingly) this very high dosage can produce alarming results - liver abnormalities, cancer, etc.

However, if we compared this dosage level to a 200 lb human, the equivalent would be .9 lbs of DHEA or over 181 bottles (25 mg., 90 count) per day or 68 capsules every hour, day and night. One would expect that this amount would not exactly be healthy for any living thing. (2.2 lbs of DHEA produces 444 bottle of 25 mg, 90 count bottles). A100 pound person, of course, would only have to take 90 bottles per day or 34 capsules per hour every hour.

# Liver Support

Even if you are using a delivery system which offers DHEA assimilation directly into the blood stream, (sublingual, spray or cream), it is recommended that you take precautions to protect the liver from any potential stress. The DHEA will still eventually travel through the liver just as all substances in the liver do, and any substance which increases the metabolic rate in the body increases the production of free radicals. The following substances have antioxidant properties and have shown to have powerful protective effects on the liver.

Alpha Lipoic Acid
Glutathione
Methionine
Silymarin

# Q&A WITH DR. RICHARD ASH

## A Comprehensive Medical Approach to Wellness with DHEA

**Q: How did you get into comprehensive medicine?**

**Ash:** I was taught to reflexively treat my patients, which is to size up the situation, put them in a category, give them a disease title and reflexively give them drugs. This is really emergency room type of medicine where drugs or surgery are used as a temporary fix for the urgent problem. I got good at using this approach and often without the side effects that a lot of physicians have, but when it came to treating myself for a type of refractory arthritis and gout, this approach didn't work. My condition was so refractory to treatment that I had to be on cortisone or prednisone therapy (20 mg. a day) for 2 1/2 years straight. I went to every expert in the world and they couldn't help me. If I lowered my dose to 19 mg. I got worse. Then I had an allergic reaction to one of the medications they put me one to lower my uric acid and almost died from just one-third the regular dosage of a drug called Alopurinol. I only took one third of the dosage because of was afraid of how I would respond, If I would have taken the full dosage, I probably wouldn't be here today. I realized through hundreds of hours of communications with various experts in alternative medicine that treating the symptoms was never going to really get me well, the cause of the problem needs to be addressed and body needs to be treated as a whole. I learned that my body was acidic and was reacting to foods and chemicals. Therefore I was refractory to treatment because of what I call our toxic load. Some things can be a burden to the body when the immune system is suppressed or overburdened. This ties in with DHEA because as any disease process continues to overwhelm the body, overload can occur which, in turn will deplete our stores of DHEA.

Immunological overload is related to our toxic burden. It's like having sand in the trunk of a perfectly good car. The extra weight is going to effect the performance of the car and may cause the engine to burn out faster. Our toxic load has an effect on our adrenal glands, which is responsible for our flight or fight response, and production of DHEA and cortisol. The body puts out cortisone and adrenaline to deal these things. Over time, the level of cortisone is depleted in the body. If you take cortisone, you are suppressing your own production of cortisone and consequently, suppressing the immune system.

After 2 1/2 years of taking prednisone, I was in a severe state and I needed to assess what was contributing to my toxic load - things in the environment, chemicals in our foods, water, etc. what nutritional deficiencies might be present. This was a large part of my recovery.

I had joint pains throughout my entire body, even if I injected cortisone directly into one joint, pain would pop up in another. This is no way to get healthy. As I began to eliminate what was contributing to my toxic load, and taking advantage of various nutritional supplements like vitamin C, etc. healing the gastrointestinal tract, and I saw the results in myself, I began to incorporate what I learned into the treatment of my patients. When they also began to improve and respond to this new form of treatment, I knew I was on to something. I started taking people off of their drugs, and striving for optimal G.I. health and soon this became the mainstay of my practice - comprehensive medicine through an alternative approach.

**Q: How did you come to use DHEA as part of your practice?**

**Ash:** I have been utilizing substances like DHEA in my practice for some time. I was introduced to DHEA by a M.D., Ph.D., who used to work at the National Institute for

Health (NIH). I was quite impressed with the results I experienced myself and wanted to pass on these potential benefits to my patients. At this time there were few physicians practicing this type of medicine so we had to use a great deal of caution, before and after testing, etc.

**Q: Why do people need to supplement DHEA?**

**Ash:** In a word, **STRESS.** We are living in a chemical world, which, without our realization, places stress upon our endocrine and immune system to the point of malfunction and illness. People today are in varying degrees of adrenal insufficiency due to immunological overload.

Imagine the burden to the body that the hundreds of chemicals in a chocolate chip cookie presents. When we drink coffee from a styrofoam cup, we can measure the styrene levels in the blood directly afterwards. This styrene can even be detected in the plague in the arteries. It's a wonder that people don't have more health problems than they do! The degree that one allows these chemicals/poisons and the type of poisons to enter the body determines our toxic load and the time period it takes immunological overload to occur. Depending on which doctor you go to, there are many different names that may be given to your condition. A rheumatologist may call it fibromyalgia, a neurologist may call it a migraine, an allergist may call it sinusitis. Many times when dealing with autoimmune diseases, (psoriasis, rheumatoid arthritis, colitis, hashimoto's, thyroiditis, MS, lupus, asthma, chronic fatigue, etc.), it can be traced to chemical sensitivities and immunological overload, and as a result, they all have excessive cortisol production in common, eventually exhausting their DHEA capacity.

The body can form antibodies and attack foods and chemicals that are present in the G.I. tract, when it shouldn't. This many times triggers the autoimmune disease to surface.

These processes cause the body to over produce cortisone and adrenaline. Low DHEA then follows as Hans Selye described as the flight or fight phenomenon. This type of stress causes low DHEA levels.

**Q: Are there warning signs that DHEA might be depressed?**

**Ash:** One of the early signs of a low DHEA is insomnia. This is due to elevated cortisol which disrupts REM sleep. At night, cortisol levels should be at there lowest when you sleep and highest when you get up in the morning.

The next sign is poor sugar regulation - hypoglycemia, where one can experience many of the symptoms of hypoglycemia - fatigue, dizziness, palpitations, headache, loss of short term memory.

The third stage is inflammation, such as joint pain, muscle aches, etc.

Finally, depression can occur where you can't even generate cortisol in the morning or at other times during the day.

These can relate to various degrees of adrenal insufficiency.

DHEA is an important part of recovery, but you also need to look at the things that are causing the problem in the first place.

**Q: What will happen if one supplements DHEA?**

**Ash:** Taking DHEA can make one feel a tremendous improvement if they were deficient before, but what we are seeing is that if the other issues that caused the adrenal insufficiency in the first place are not addressed, eventually, the other symptoms will return. You can't continue to eat glass when you are trying to heal the GI tract. You need to figure out what your "glass" is. Avoid the things that are overloading the immune system. It may be dust, mold, pollen, perfume, sulfites, pesticides, various chemicals, and even foods such as wheat, corn, milk, chocolate, etc., until you are recovered. You may not have to eliminate all of these things forever, but healing will be impeded if you don't.

Think of the body as a biological bank account. You want to build up the reserves and decrease the spending. The spending is wasting energy unnecessarily, such as putting in chemicals and substances in the body producing unnecessary hypersensitivity reactions.

There are various ways in which we can test for these sensitivities that we can do to determine many of these, all which we use to identify the foods and/or chemicals which are the culprit causing hypersensitivity reactions.

### Q: So you are saying that DHEA is just acting as a temporary fix?

**Ash:** Unless the other underlying issues are addressed, yes, DHEA is only a temporary fix. If there are electrical shorts in the wiring of the battery in your car or if the alternator (which charges your battery) is not working, eventually, that will place a drain on the battery. If you charge it it will be OK for that day, but eventually you will be somewhere and you won't be able to start your car because you didn't get at the cause of the problem.

### Q: What can happen?

**Ash:** People will get to the point that they have DHEA depletion and adrenal insufficiency and they are totally resistant to therapy. In the long term, people could be doing harm to themselves by taking DHEA and not addressing the cause of their problems.

There are a lot of so-called foods on the market which is actually just a bunch of chemicals that taste good (at least to some people) that these can become just as dangerous as some of the drugs on the market, because people think they are harmless, yet there is no regulation.

Many people are taking DHEA at dosages higher than what they need. This can cause side effects in the short term (acne, headaches, irritability, sleep problems. hair growth in women, etc.) but in the long term can alter their endocrine balance.

Most people do not monitor their DHEA or other hormone levels with before and after tests. Saliva testing can accurate, very affordable, and convenient.

The key to DHEA and hormone replacement is balance and harmony. More is not better. Our immune system is like an orchestra. Biochemical reactions occur optimally with the proper concentrations of ingredients in the mix. Too much water also can be harmful, like anything else.

In regards to side effects - dangers - There can actually be much more serious dangers of **NOT** taking DHEA if you need it then to take DHEA in the proper amount. Proper amount is the key. If you are low in DHEA and your DHEA/cortisol levels are off, and you do not do anything about it, you can wind up with chronic immunosuppression and ultimately can be some of the underlying reasons for increasing the potential risk of cancer. Immunosuppression results from Interleuken-2 suppression which is discussed in detail earlier in the book.

Remember, DHEA can help us deal with stress, but too much DHEA can create anxiety and diminishes our ability to deal with stress as a possible side effect.

**Q: Do you feel DHEA should be regulated as a prescription drug?**

**Ash:** I do, because DHEA should only given to those individuals who need it. I do not recommend it to individuals who come to me requesting it that do not have test results which indicate it's need. Blood tests will measure the bound fraction, whereas I like to measure the free faction which is measured by a saliva test. I also like to measure cortisol levels four different times throughout the day. This is difficult to do with a blood test because the person has to go back to the lab four different times. The saliva samples can be collected without difficulty with the sample collection materials they can take with them.

Cortisol secretion by the adrenal glands fluctuates

throughout the day. It should be the highest in the morning, lowest during the night allowing one to fall into REM sleep, but if one is hypoglycemic, for example, one will continue to produce high amounts through the night and inhibit one's ability to get a good nights sleep. These are the types of things one needs to examine before prescribing DHEA.

**Q: Besides taking too much, what other mistakes do people make with DHEA supplementation?**

**Ash:** What most people do not do on their own, meaning without the care of a physician, is to ensure that their cortisol levels are coming down as they are increasing their DHEA. Cortisol levels via saliva testing should be no more than 3 at 11-12 at night. If if is higher than this, there is not a chance that they are going to get a good nights sleep. There are nutrients such as phosphatidylserine that can be used to help bring down cortisol levels. One needs to be aware of what their cortical levels are throughout the day because if cortisol levels are normal in the morning, around 13, one does not want to take a cortisol lowering agent. Phosphatidylserine, for example, is often sold on the market as a brain/memory enhancing supplement, so one would think that it would be good to take in the morning, but it could lower cortisol when you don't want it to.

Cortisol levels of some people measures 50 (when it should never be higher than 23 in the morning and never higher than 3 at night), four times per day. They are putting out so much cortisol that they are in a chronic hyper state and the body is continually putting out cortisol and adrenaline, cortisol and adrenaline. We want to regulate the blood sugar because when one is eating a high sugar diet the body falls into a cycle of increased blood sugar, increased insulin, etc. One thing to do is eat foods which have a low glycemic index.

When blood sugar is low the brain produces neurotransmitters which tell you you are hungry. Your brain decides what to eat. Each food we eat effects us in a different way. Some foods are more satisfying than others. An apple may be more sugar stabilizing than a chocolate chip cookie, even though they have approximately the same number of calories. Sometimes you can eat something, feel satisfied and then be hungry again in 50 minutes.

When you eat something, as your blood sugar rises, insulin is released transporting glucose into the cells. Some foods cause the blood sugar level to increase more quickly and to a higher level than others. A dramatic rise in blood sugar corresponds to a dramatic rise in insulin, and many more times a rapid fall of glucose.

Glycemic index is a rating system indicating how different foods effect the rise in blood sugar and the consequent trigger of insulin secretion. Foods which have such a dramatic effect on blood sugar are rated higher. Reactions are compared to table sugar, which is rated 100, which has the most dramatic effect of sugar levels.

*Low glycemic index* foods promote a slow, moderate rise in blood sugar and insulin after eating them. This helps keep hunger in check and encourage the body to dissolve body fat by converting it into energy. These foods allow you to consume more calories without gaining weight. They can actually increase your metabolic rate. Lower insulin levels promote maximum fat breakdown as compared to higher insulin levels which can promote fat synthesis and storage.

*High glycemic index* foods cause sudden, unstable swings in blood sugar, first with rapid, very high sugar and insulin surges, followed by a crash of sugar to excessively low levels. These foods increase your cravings for simple carbohydrates, sweets, etc., causing overeating and binging. **(See pages 226-227 for a glycemic index.)**

**Q: Some people like to use DHEA because of the effects they feel such as increased energy, increased sex drive, etc. can you comment on this?**

**Ash:** There are certainly things that are available to up regulate yourself, but they are always at a cost. Balance is the key and when you start messing with the system, without considering the body's feedback mechanisms, you can get into trouble down the line. For example, if you take cortisone, the body is going to stop producing its own cortisone, this is why it should only be prescribed for short intervals at a time, if at all since there are alternative choices available.

For those who are using DHEA to treat an acute condition such as an asthma attack or allergies, this is not how I prefer to use DHEA. Instead I would like to treat the patient so that these attacks are prevented. DHEA may be part of this treatment, but it would include powdered pharmaceutical grade buffered vitamin C with quercetin or OPC. I start patients out at with a few thousand milligrams four times a day. To determine proper individual dosage this may be increased to bowel tolerance and then decreased by 25%. It has been as high as 200,000 grams in certain individuals. It is different for each person depending on their individual situation. This regulates and decreases inflammation in the GI tract and stimulates the immune system for defense and repair immediately. Many allergic responses are due to GI tract dysbiosis.

I want to add that after a period of time, as the body responds positively, one may decrease their intake accordingly.

Some men can be impotent because they have low DHEA levels. If I gave them testosterone shots if can take care of the problem temporarily, but it would be better to give them DHEA and deal directly with the source of the problem. Some DHEA can convert to testosterone and their sex drive can be improved.

**Q: Do you recommend Pregnenolone supplementation in addition to DHEA?**

**Ash:** In some cases pregnenolone is indicated in conjunction to or in place of DHEA. For example, if I want to lower DHEA because of side effects such as acne, anxiety, headaches, etc. I will prescribe 10 to a total 100 mg Pregnenolone.

Pregnenolone can convert to antiinflammatory cortisone or progesterone.

**Q: What about prostate cancer?**

**Ash:** It is a difficult situation when a male patient is low in DHEA, but has a positive PSA (prostate specific antigen) which is a screen for cancer. I first get PSA's on all men who I am placing on DHEA. If one has a positive PSA, I then do a PSA I (indicates enlargement) and PSA II (indicates possible cancer) to determine the cause. As DHEA could increase one's levels of testosterone which could accelerate the growth of prostate cancer, therefore, as a precaution, DHEA is contraindicated in patients with prostate cancer.

**Q: Can too much DHEA (supplemental) contribute to ovarian cysts or fibroids?**

**Ash:** I do not recommend DHEA capsules because of the higher rate of conversion to estrogens which could aggravate such conditions, and also others such as women with a history of breast cancer, endometriosis, cervical cancer, dysplasia, etc. If tests show that DHEA levels are low, I would recommend DHEA sublingual, **NOT** capsules. Pregnenolone is sometimes preferred in addition to low intake of DHEA, or preferred in certain situations.

**Q: Do you recommend DHEA for patients with chronic fatigue?**

**Ash:** It depends on their test results. If their test indicate that they need it, and I already know that they are in stage 3, 4, or 5 of adrenal insufficiency, I would recommend the sublingual or the spray. I generally do not recommend capsules at all any more.

**Q: What effects on the liver does one need to concern themselves with?**

**Ash:** I have not run into any problems with patients experiencing liver problems. Problems would only be to what I would deem to be miss- use of DHEA, that is, taking DHEA at very high doses.

According to Dr. Rao, Department of Pathology at Northwestern Medical School in Chicago, who did extensive testing on laboratory rats with very high levels of DHEA to assess the effects on the liver. He did find effects on the peroxisome enzymes, but concluded that the application did not apply to humans as the study results were species specific. Also, they used such an incredibly high dosage on the animals (according to body weight) that you could not compare the results they had to any possible effect to humans.

**Q: Can you comment on the various delivery systems of DHEA, side effects, disadvantages, advantages of each, etc.?**

**Ash:** I started out using capsules (5 mg. or 10 mg. one to two times per day up to a maximum of 25 mg. total for men only) on my patients but I was unhappy because we didn't get the absorption that we were looking for, largely because it must first be absorbed from the GI tract and then had to pass through the liver before it got to the blood stream. Certain individuals had gastrointestinal side effects to the capsules,

When using 25 and 50 mg. capsules, certain people were experiencing side effects off too much conversion to testosterone which can cause acne, headaches, vaginal spotting, breast tenderness, and even some gastrointestinal problems.

Next I tried the transdermal gel where the hormone is absorbed through the skin just like an estrogen patch. We saw better absorption, it eliminated the gastrointestinal problems and we were able to keep the dosage low; 7 mg. for men twice per day and 3-5 mg. for women twice a day. The disadvantage of this delivery system is that the hormone can remain in the fat cells a little too long. Also, one can get too much conversion to estrogen and/or testosterone which many times is undesirable. I always did before and after levels to check the effects.

In women, the best way to check their monthly curve of hormonal production is with a protocol evaluation which requires saliva samples every two to three days for a whole month. This gives us a much better idea what is really going on as it is much more accurate than just checking levels on any given day.

With the Progest™ cream I was seeing toxic levels of progesterone because it remained bound in the fat cells. Instead of having a normal level of under 100, I saw levels over 1,000. Even after women stopped using the cream for six months, the level would only drop from 1,000 to 870. The DHEA or Pregnenolone creams are not as bad because they can convert to the other hormones, unlike the progesterone in Progest™.

I prefer to recommend DHEA before recommending female hormone replacement therapy. I prefer the liquid sublingual DHEA (1 to 5 mg. per drop). This delivery system allows the DHEA to go straight into the blood stream avoiding the liver. There is also less conversion to estrogen and testosterone.

**Q: What results are you seeing in your patients?**

**Ash:** Following are examples of patients treated successfully at the Ash Center for Comprehensive Medicine. Each situation is different and therefore warrants a different protocol. To begin, the adrenal function of each patient was assessed with an Adrenal Stress Test and Temporal Adrenal Profile, measuring free cortisol levels (nM) at four different times by saliva collection and analysis. Note the normal ranges for each time period.

**Normal Cortisol Range**

| | |
|---|---|
| **7:00-8:00 AM** | **13-23** |
| **11:00-12:00 PM** | **4-8** |
| **4:00-5:00 PM** | **3-8** |
| **11:00-11:59PM** | **1-3** |

**Cortisol Time Integral: 23-42**

Cortisol levels should be highest in the morning. This is what wakes us up and gives us motivation. At night, cortisol levels should be lowest so we are relaxed, able to go to sleep. enter REM stage of sleep, stay asleep and and actually get a good night's rest.

**DHEA& DHEA(S): Normal range is between 3-10 mg/ml**

## <u>Key for DHEA-Cortisol Correlation</u>

**Stage 1**. Stress adapted "hyper" response, minimal change

**Stage 2**. Stress adapted with a divergence in response to ACTH

**Stage 3.** Maladaptation Phase 1

**Stage 4.** Maladaptation Phase 2

**Stage 5.** Adrenal fatigue, non-adapted

**Stage 6.** Inappropriate DHEAS with non ACTH dependent stimulation

**Stage 7.** Adrenal failure

## Patient #1

Female, age 44
Symptoms: Fatigue, insomnia, allergies, headaches, GI complaints such as constipation, diarrhea, gas, bloating, etc.

|                    | **Before**      | **After**          |
|--------------------|-----------------|--------------------|
| **7:00-8:00 AM**   | **39** (Elevated) | **16** (Normal)   |
| **11:00-12:00 PM** | **11** (Elevated) | **8** (Normal)    |
| **4:00-5:00 PM**   | **83** (Elevated) | **6** (Normal)    |
| **11:00-11:59PM**  | **63** (Elevated) | **5** (Slightly elev.) |

| | | |
|---|---|---|
| **Cortisol Time Integral: 196** (Elevated) | **35** (Normal) |
| **DHEA& DHEA(S)** | **3** (Borderline) | **5** (Borderline) |
| **DHEA-Cortisol correlation:  Stage 2-3** | **Normal** |

*Ash Comments and Recommendations:* This patient was placed on our standard protocol of DHEA, Phosphatidylserine to lower cortisol which was very high, especially at night which was causing the insomnia. Also part of our standard protocol are pure Vitamin C (to bowel tolerance, less 25%*), Quercetin and other bioflavonoids, OPC, amino acids, a multivitamin, other vitamins, a low glycemic index diet and other stress reducing practices, etc. You can see how she responded nicely with normal cortisol, DHEA and adrenal function.

*\* Vitamin C bowel tolerance varies a great deal from person to person. Pure vitamin C is given in increased quantities until the patient experiences loose stools. This amount is then reduced by 25%. As health improves over time, the need for vitamin C decreases as reserves are restored.*

## Patient #2

Male, age 44
Symptoms: Sinusitis, allergies, eczema, GI disturbances such as bloating and gas, memory problems, etc.

|  | **Before** | **After** |
|---|---|---|
| **7:00-8:00 AM** | **70** (Elevated) | **22** (Normal) |
| **11:00-12:00 PM** | **10** (Elevated) | **16** (Elevated) |
| **4:00-5:00 PM** | **30** (Elevated) | **9** (Borderline) |
| **11:00-11:59PM** | **12** (Elevated) | **3** (Normal) |
| **Cortisol Time Integral: 122** (Elevated) | | **50** (Slightly elev.) |
| **DHEA& DHEA(S)** **2** (Depressed) | | **7** (Normal) |
| **DHEA-Cortisol correlation: Stage 3** | | **Stage 2** |

*Ash Comments and Recommendations:* This individual's symptoms improved greatly with our standard protocol of DHEA, Phosphatidylserine, Vitamin C, etc. This person also has a problem of heavy metal toxicity and went through chelation treatment which he responded favorably to.

**Patient #3**

Female, age 45
Symptoms: Lyme Disease, fibromyalgia, chronic fatigue

|  | **Before** | **After** |
|---|---|---|
| **7:00-8:00 AM** | 81(Elevated) | 17 (Normal) |
| **11:00-12:00 PM** | 12 (Elevated) | 16 (Elevated) |
| **4:00-5:00 PM** | 13 (Elevated) | 8 (Normal) |
| **11:00-11:59PM** | 10 (Elevated) | 5 (Elevated) |
| **Cortisol Time Integral:** 116 (Elevated) | | 44 (Slightly Elev.) |
| **DHEA& DHEA(S)** 3 (Borderline) | | 6 (Normal) |
| **DHEA-Cortisol correlation: Stage 3** | | **Stage 1** |

*Ash Comments and Recommendations:* This individual had been to a number of infectious disease specialists without experiencing improvement. We were able to improve her adrenal status, restore her cortisol and DHEA to normal. In addition to DHEA, we used intravenous vitamin and mineral therapy and other more aggressive treatments to improve her energy levels, sleep, and etc.

**Patient #4**

Female, age 53
Symptoms: Menopausal symptoms, headaches, depression, chronic fatigue, insomnia, irritable, angry.

|                | Before | After |
|----------------|--------|-------|
| **7:00-8:00 AM** | 6 (Depressed) | 69 (Elevated) |
| **11:00-12:00 PM** | 12 (Elevated) | 60 (Elevated) |
| **4:00-5:00 PM** | 13 (Elevated) | 10 (Elevated) |
| **11:00-11:59PM** | 7 (Elevated) | 9 (Elevated) |

| | | |
|---|---|---|
| **Cortisol Time Integral: 38** (Elevated) | | **148** (Elevated) |
| **DHEA& DHEA(S)** 2 (Depressed) | | **2** (Depressed) |
| **DHEA-Cortisol correlation: Stage 3** | | **Stage 3** |

*Ash Comments and Recommendations*: She was taking a number of medications for her depression and insomnia. I put her on DHEA and a number of other things and although she is still is stage 3, her adrenal function is improving and her symptoms and state of mind greatly improved. She is laughing and feeling much better. Before she couldn't even produce enough cortisol to get out of bed in the morning. She was at the stage where she needed physiological cortisol to rest the adrenal glands.

**Patient #5**

Female, age 50
Symptoms: Hives, allergies, insomnia.

|  | **Before** | **After** |
|---|---|---|
| **7:00-8:00 AM** | 32 (Elevated) | 36 (Elevated) |
| **11:00-12:00 PM** | 14 (Elevated) | 19 (Elevated) |
| **4:00-5:00 PM** | 10 (Elevated) | 12 (Elevated) |
| **11:00-11:59PM** | 7 (Elevated) | 6 (Slightly elev.) |

| | | |
|---|---|---|
| **Cortisol Time Integral:** 63 (Elevated) | | 73 (Elevated) |
| **DHEA& DHEA(S)** 2 (Depressed) | | 4 (Borderline) |
| **DHEA-Cortisol correlation:** Stage 3 | | Stage 2 |

*Ash Comments and Recommendations:* Hives and environmental sensitivities are very difficult to treat because you must determine what they are and then eliminate them until they can be tolerated. In this case, she was reactive to almost everything we tested her for. She had major improvements in her symptoms as she responded to the DHEA, phosphatidlyserine, intravenous vitamin C, etc.

**Patient #6**

Female, age 63
Symptoms: Diabetic, circulation problems,insomnia, fatigue.

|  | **Before** | **After** |
|---|---|---|
| **7:00-8:00 AM** | 81 (Elevated) | 70 (Elevated) |
| **11:00-12:00 PM** | 84 (Elevated) | 66 (Elevated) |
| **4:00-5:00 PM** | 40 (Elevated) | 9 (Borderline) |
| **11:00-11:59PM** | 86 (Elevated) | 5 (Elevated) |
| **Cortisol Time Integral:** | 291 (Elevated) | 150 (Slightly elev.) |
| **DHEA& DHEA(S)** | 3 (Depressed) | 2 (Depressed) |
| **DHEA-Cortisol correlation:** | Stage 3 | Stage 3 |

*Ash Comments and Recommendations:* In addition to our standard protocol, this patient was given chelation for her circulatory problems. Her symptoms did improve. We lowered her cortisol, especially at night so she was able to sleep better, but because of diabetic condition and some other problems her overall adrenal function did not change,

**Patient #7**

Female, age 45
Symptoms: Irritable bowel, hypothyroid, degenerative joint disease,

|  | **Before** | **After** |
|---|---|---|
| **7:00-8:00 AM** | 12 (Depressed) | 11 (Depressed) |
| **11:00-12:00 PM** | 11 (Elevated) | 8 (Normal) |
| **4:00-5:00 PM** | 12 (Elevated) | 6 (Normal) |
| **11:00-11:59PM** | 7 (Elevated) | 3 (Normal) |
| **Cortisol Time Integral:** 42 (Elevated) | | 28 (Normal.) |
| **DHEA& DHEA(S)** | 1 (Depressed) | 4 (Normal) |
| **DHEA-Cortisol correlation:  Stage 3** | | **Normal** |

*Ash Comments and Recommendations:* This individuals responded quickly with our standard protocol.

# HOW TO MAINTAIN AND NATURALLY RAISE HEALTHY DHEA LEVELS

*Researchers have discovered that living a sensible healthy lifestyle pays off in the long run! For example, they found that a 45 year-old man who followed few or no "healthy habits" could expect about 21.6 additional years, while someone who followed six or seven could expect to live 33 more years. Even doing something as simple as eating breakfast, and getting enough sleep added more than 11 years to a man's life. By comparison, having both sets of parents and grand parents live to age 80 increases one's life expectancy by only about 3 years.*

*The trend held good for older age groups as well. If someone followed all seven good habits, his health at age 75 was comparable to that of someone in his 30s or 40s who neglected good habits.*

There are a number of ways to naturally increase the DHEA levels in your body no matter what age you are:

## 1. Increase exercise and exercise on a regular basis.

Exercise is one of the best natural ways to increase DHEA levels in men and women. Higher levels of muscle tissue in the body boost testosterone levels. This may be one of the reasons that men have higher DHEA levels compared to women. Exercise also helps reduce stress, which is known to decrease DHEA levels.

## 2. Do not smoke and avoid others who smoke.

Smoking depresses hormone production and hormone function in the body. Nicotine, among its many other negative effects in the body, mimics iodine, effecting functioning of the thyroid gland and entire endocrine system.

## 3. Avoid alcohol or drink only in moderation.

Alcohol puts an added stress on the body. Alcohol has numerous and various effects on hormone production in the the body. Female heavy drinkers have been found to have lower DHEA-S levels (39 percent lower), higher testosterone levels and lower progesterone levels than non drinking controls.

## 4. Avoid synthetic steroid hormone analogs.

Taking synthetic analogs depresses our natural hormone production and hormone function in the body. Synthetic hormones taken on a daily basis for an extended period, such as birth control pills or for hormone replacement therapy, can cause the most harm.

## 5. Avoid stress and practice relaxation.

Chronic stress and stressful events have a harsh effect on the adrenal glands and can depress DHEA production as much as 50 percent.

Find ways to reduce or deal with stress such as exercise, spend time with family, friends, pets, etc., attend church, meditate, pray, sing, play a musical instrument, listen to relaxing music or find some other way to obtain inner peace and relaxation. Laugh. Enjoy each day. Have a fresh, optimistic outlook on life!

To prevent stress and aging of the skin (and skin cancer):

Avoid the sun, avoid the sun, and avoid the sun! Use a minimum of SPF 15, especially on the face, if you are going to be outdoors. Wear a hat and protective clothing.

## 6. Get adequate amounts of sleep each night.

Sleep deprivation puts a tremendous amount of stress on the body making us susceptible to ill health. During sleep the body heals, grows, and recovers. Keeping a regular schedule also puts less stress on the body.

## 7. Maintain ideal weight.

Determine what your ideal weight is according to your bone structure, height, sex, and other factors. Maintain normal weight - i.e., not more than 5 percent under weight, and no more than 10 percent overweight for women, and not more than 20 percent overweight for men.)

Don't pay too much attention to those insurance type weight charts which allow you to gain weight as you get older. These charts also don't take in consideration the fact that muscle weighs more than fat. According to their calculations, most athletic muscular individuals are overweight.

## 8. Keep body fat percentage low.

Decreased body fat is strongly correlated with increased DHEA levels. Healthy body fat percentages for men range from approximately 5-12%, for women, 14-21%.

## 9. Eat a healthy, well balanced diet.

● Substitute meat protein with fish, beans or other low fat sources of protein. Soy beans provide complete protein nutrition. Soy milk is nutritious, good tasting, requires no refrigeration and can be stored indefinitely. Fish contains oils that may prevent heart attacks. Heart disease is the number one cause of death in the U.S.

● Eat plenty of fruits and vegetables which are loaded with phytonutrients and antioxidants proven to protect us against cancer and many other degenerative diseases. Foods high in beta carotenes (carrots, spinach, broccoli, cantaloupe). Beta carotene is protective against cancer - the number two cause of death in the US.

● Avoid refined foods, sugar and chemical additives to food. Eat more complex carbohydrates

● Eat a high fiber diet.

● Eat a low-fat diet. Avoid fried foods, saturated fat (i.e., tropical oils) and hydrogenated oils. Read labels before buying and make ingredient inquiries when eating out! Instead use unsaturated oils such as found in fish, flax seeds and olive oil.

● Eat foods high in vitamin C (citrus, green vegetables, green peppers, etc.).

● Eat foods high in vitamin E (vegetable oils and grains), zinc (mushrooms, oysters, pumpkin seeds), and selenium (bran, tuna, fish).

● Drink distilled water or use an effective filtering device.

## 10. Utilize supplements when necessary.
Be sure you are obtaining adequate amounts of vitamins, minerals, amino acids, essential fatty acids, to prevent defi-

ciencies which create susceptibility to numerous disease conditions.

Osteoporosis, heart disease, hypoglycemia, many types of cancer and other numerous disease conditions are directly or closely associated with dietary and nutritional factors. Most all disease conditions are associated with low DHEA levels. If you can prevent the disease through nutritional means, you may be able to help keep your DHEA levels elevated.

If you are uncomfortable with the idea of taking pre-formed free form DHEA or DHEA-S, take wild yam. Not everyone is efficient in converting phytochemical precursors in diosgenin to hormones such as progesterone; however, there are many advantages because the body will only make as much as it needs.

Diosgenin has shown to increase levels of hormones such as progesterone when taken orally and/or applied transdermally. There are no known side effects of diosgenin extracted from wild yams compared to using synthetic analog hormones.

# FREQUENTLY ASKED QUESTIONS ABOUT DHEA:

*Q: Isn't DHEA only available through prescription?*

*A:* Prior to October 1994 when the Health and Education Act of 1994 went into effect, DHEA was not available over the counter. This law changed the status of DHEA and it is now considered a *natural substance,* for which no prescription is required. Again, no prescription is required for freeform DHEA. To my knowledge, DHEA-Sulfate (DHEA-S), which is a compound, is still only available through a prescription and a compounding pharmacist who can make it.

*Q: What is the difference between DHEA-S and freeform DHEA?*

*A.* In DHEA-S free-form DHEA is compounded with a sulfate molecule. This sulfate allows the body to metabolize the DHEA at a slower rate (referred to as "half-life" in the body). For example, if you are taking two 25 mg capsules per day of free form DHEA it is recommended that you take one in the am and one in the pm to maintain a steady level. With DHEA-S one could take both capsules at once and maintain a steady level.

The half-life of freeform DHEA capsules is from 8 to 13 hours. The half-life of DHEA-S is closer to 20 hours. Otherwise, in the body there really is no difference. They are used interchangeably.

*Q: Is DHEA a drug?*

*A:* It is not considered a drug. DHEA is a natural substance. Natural substances cannot be patented - which was largely the reason that no companies were manufacturing it in the U.S. Throughout Europe it has been used for some time for it's anti-aging and health promoting benefits.

DHEA is considered a semi-synthetic because it is processed from a natural sterol base. It is <u>not</u> an analog like many of the prescription synthetic hormones, like medroprogesterone acetate progestins, and conjugated estrogen tablets (such as Premarin®). These are not the same exact chemical as those we manufacture in our bodies. The free form DHEA now available without a prescription is pure chemical DHEA, it is exactly like the DHEA manufactured by our own adrenal glands.

### Q: How is free form DHEA made?

*A:* The sterol base used by the laboratories manufacturing free form DHEA is a non-animal cholesterol. All hormones in the body are made from cholesterol. The source for this non-animal cholesterol could be any vegetable sterol, such as soy.

### Q: Is wild yam used to make DHEA?

*A:* There are currently two DHEA manufactures using wild yam as the raw material to produce DHEA. A third company uses soy, a fourth uses rice. Plant sterols can be obtained from a number of sources.

### Q: Does DHEA have any negative effects?

*A:* Not if it is used to simply to replenish your levels to the point when they were highest. In men, over age 45, this would be around 50 mg.; in women, about 25 mg. Most of the clinical studies conducted over the last several years which I researched for my book, used 50 mg. capsules. This amount was found to be very safe and effective in healthy individuals. Many practitioners including Dr. Regelson and Dr. Ash, recommend a lower dosage.

Individuals who have serious health problems may require higher levels but I would strongly suggest that these individuals be under the care of a physician who is familiar with using

DHEA for therapeutic purposes.

Taking very, very high levels of DHEA over a prolonged period has been shown to create liver abnormalities. But, remember, too much aspirin can be very harmful. Too much of *anything* can be harmful.

Excess amounts in women can be detected by the appearance of facial hair. Headaches and irritability are also indications that you are taking more than you need in men and women.

**Q: *Does a person under the age of 30 need to take DHEA?***

**A:** It depends on the state of one's health. If someone is perfectly healthy, has minimal stress, and doesn't smoke or drink, and exercises on a regular basis, I would say probably not. After the age of 40, however, most people can experience benefits.

If one has a chronic medical problem, at any age, DHEA, used properly, can be extremely beneficial. One can easily determine if they can benefit by DHEA supplementation by taking a DHEA saliva test.

**Q: *Are natural products safer and more effective than the actual synthesized product?***

**A:** Natural products are far safer than using synthetic analogs. Whenever the body can be encouraged to help itself, it is far better. You want to achieve balance in the body, not stress. Synthetic hormone analogs actually create stress in the body because they are not exactly the same substance as what the body produces. They may produce similar results, but with side effects. Also, introducing synthetic hormone analogs into the body throws off the balance of all the other hormones. This doesn't happen with Dioscorea or with DHEA taken properly.

With synthetic hormones, dosage cycling is very important because cycling is the natural process for the body. If you suddenly stop taking the hormone or if you continue to take the hormone for an extended period of time there will be problems. You can easily create a situation with synthetics where you cause the adrenals to shut down or a number of other side effects can result. This frequently happens with cortisone and other synthetic hormones.

There is no evidence demonstrating that precursors are as effective as synthesized DHEA when taken in the proper amounts. In some situations, particularly in the case of bone restoration, precursors may be just as effective.

Any time a substance, natural or synthetic, can make a change in the body, for example, heal, act as an anti-inflammatory, or an antibacterial, etc., the possibility exists for side effects. Because so many pharmaceutical chemical compounds are so dangerous, the American public is now rushing toward alternative therapies to avoid side effects.

The Hippocratic Oath states, *"First, do no harm."*

For the most part, side effects are not intentional and there are many life-saving pharmaceutical compounds in existence. There is a balance to seek between allopathic medicine and natural/ herbal/preventative medicine. There are many natural substances which will give us the responses we are looking for with fewer side effects. We should be utilize these substances more often.

**Q: *Does yam extract actually convert into DHEA, estrogens and progesterone in the body?***

**A:** Phyto-precursors provided in wild yam have been providing women with an alternative to synthetic analogs for some time. Wild yam has been recommended for women's problems because of the high amounts of diosgenin which is very similar to progesterone in the body. The yam extract may not convert into progesterone, but because the molecular structure is so similar between the two, the body may be able to use it like it was progesterone. From progesterone the body can make estrogens or any number of other hormones.

There is no published clinical evidence to show that diosgenin converts to DHEA in the body. While the body is a brilliant chemical manufacturing plant, it has a reduced ability to manufacture DHEA as we grow older. The ability to convert such a substance as diosgenin to DHEA is likely to diminish as well (if we actually have that ability at all).

I have heard from reputable doctors such as Dr. Bob Martin of the popular radio talk show, *Health Talk*, based out of Phoenix, AZ., that he has seen patients increase their DHEA levels while taking fairly high dosages of a wild yam extract product (9 tablets daily). He found that not all brands of wild yam extract had this effect. He also told me that that particular brand did not have that effect in everyone, even at high dosages.

DHEA researchers like Dr. Neecie Moore have reported similar findings.

Natural substances usually do not have the dramatic effect that synthetic drugs do. This is one of the reasons that they don't have side effects. There is really no way to determine how much wild yam extract would be required to obtain the same effects. We really don't know if this is a possibility, we just don't have enough information to answer all of the questions. More research is needed.

Some organizations such as CERI have clearly stated that *"...according to published literature, the human body cannot convert phytosterols into pregnenolone. And without pregnenolone, the body cannot make DHEA."* (Smart Drug News, February 29, 1996, pg 12.)

However, remember the Diosgenin molecule is very similar to the progesterone molecule and there is a greater potential that women will experience progesterone benefits.

The food sources we ingest, both good and bad, are used by the body in many different ways. Many of the chemicals we ingest ultimately end up as carcinogens. A lot of these phytochemicals and phytosterols are very similar to pharmaceuticals, which is really what stimulated the interest in synthesizing the material from them.

The human body has an amazing ability to heal itself if given the chance. The American consumer is demanding information concerning how to do this. Many are seeking alternative therapies which could possibly save our health care systems both from an efficiency standpoint as well as a financial one.

It would be very difficult to absorb enough diosgenin to reach levels required for therapeutic purposes. In addition, if you already have a medical problem, it would be unlikely that the body could convert diosgenin to DHEA at all. If you are interested in treating a medical condition, I would suggest that you contact a physician who is familiar with using free form DHEA or DHEA-S in this manner.

If you are uncomfortable with the idea of taking preformed free form DHEA or DHEA-S, take wild yam. Not everyone is efficient in converting phytochemical precursors to DHEA; however, there are many advantages because the body would only make as much as it needs.

**Q: Is there a risk that the body will shut down its natural production of DHEA if one takes supplemental DHEA for a prolonged period?**

**A:** Not when taken at low so called "anti-aging" or "preventative" doses. For women, 30 to 50 years old, this is about 5 to 25 mg, for women over age 50, 5 to 50 mg. encapsulated

For men, 30 to 50 years old this is between 10 to 50 mg, and for men over age 50, 25 to 75 mg. encapsulated.

If taking amounts higher than this, I would recommend first cutting back on the dose for a few days before stopping to prevent any sudden changes. After this, the body should go back to the amount it would normally produce for someone your age, sex and state of health.

Some researchers, such as Dr. William Regelson, have suggested alternate day dosages for any long term corticosteriod treatment to help prevent any type of adrenal problems. However, DHEA is not the same as cortisone. DHEA levels decrease with age, but cortisone levels remain stable or even increase with age.

Some physicians who prescribe DHEA for therapeutic purposes suggest cycling, such as taking a week off after being on a daily regimen for three weeks.

Some researchers have found that very high doses and long term use of the prescription form of DHEA capsules may weaken the adrenal glands - similar to the effects (although to a milder extent) of cortisone. However, Dr. Ash and other experts believe that the liquid sublingual is generally overall much safer than capsules.

### Q: *Does one need to take DHEA forever?*

**A:** If you want to continue to enjoy the benefits of taking it. One should want to continue taking a safe, low "anti-aging" dose indefinitely. If using therapeutic doses, it is conceivable that individuals could gradually improve their condition and strengthen their bodies to the point where a a lower dosage could be utilized over time. A higher dose could be used to treat symptoms as needed.

### Q: *Can DHEA supplements increase sexual desire and functioning in both men and women?*

**A:** Because of the many different effects that DHEA has in the body, it would seem normal that sexual desire would increase in both men and women. DHEA supplementation generally slows down the aging process, increases energy, and can increase levels of estrogen in women and testosterone in men, often to levels found in younger men and women.

Testimonials in this book and elsewhere in DHEA literature, reveal a normalization or enhancement of sexual desire and functioning even in older men and women in many cases.

**Q:** *Can menstrual periods which have ceased to occur due to menopause start again when taking DHEA or progesterone supplements?*

**A:** Even in women who have gone through menopause, breakthrough bleeding can occur temporarily due to increased levels of progesterone combined with the release of excess stored estrogens in the female. This should cease in a few days, and definitely in a matter of a few months. If it does not, you should contact your physician.

If, however, a woman had entered menopause prematurely due to stress, drug use or other unnatural cause, menstrual periods may return to a regular cycle after the adrenal glands and endocrine system normalizes. It may be inconvenient, but it is natural. DHEA "turns back the clock" in many people. However, if you are well past menopausal age and menses still continues, you should consult your physician.

**Q:** *If a women has been on synthetic hormones (estrogen and/or progestins) for a long time, can she stop taking them if she takes DHEA and progesterone precursors?*

**A:** DHEA does increase natural estrogen and progesterone levels. Natural progesterone from diosgenins extracted from certain wild yam species also increase progesterone levels.

Many, well-respected physicians, including John Lee, M.D., Robert Atkins, M.D., Julian Whitaker, M.D., as well as Betty Kamen, Ph.D., have reported that women can safely avoid dangerous synthetic hormones and even get better results in reducing hot flashes, PMS, osteoporosis, cardiovascular disease and cancer, and increasing libido using DHEA and natural progesterone. The F.D.A., F.T.C. and drug companies are sure to fight this, but the facts of clinical experience over the past few years shows that in most cases, side effects of synthetic hormones outweigh their benefits.

Dr. David Williams, editor of the highly respected newsletter "*Alternatives*" and renowned expert in non-invasive and natural therapies, states that natural progesterone may eliminate the need for synthetic estrogen in the prevention of the bone thinning disease and osteoporosis, which is responsible for 1.3 million bone fractures in women over age 45. According to Dr. Williams, clinical studies have shown that all post menopausal women, age 38-83 using cream with natural hormone compounds from wild yams increased bone density levels. Some increased their density levels as much as 25 percent. So, unlike synthetic estrogens, which only slow down bone loss, these natural compounds actually restore bone density with no dangerous side effects.

It may be advisable to switch to a lower dosage of the synthetic hormones before stopping taking them all together. As always, check with your physician and share with him or her the information in this book.

**Q:** *Can hormone imbalances be attributed to our diet or environment?*

**A:** Only in the last few years have we begun to see the impact of outside influences upon our hormone levels. We know that smoking and alcohol affect our hormones. We know that a diet which is very high in fat and highly processed foods containing chemicals and chemical residues affects our hormone levels. These contaminants are not only in our food, they are also in the water and air. We absorb these chemicals. You can be assured that they affect us, and not much good can come of it. Pesticides and petrochemicals are fat soluble and have characteristics similar to estrogen in the body. They are actually pseudo - estrogens. Excess estrogens and pseudo-estrogens are deposited in fatty tissue such as the breasts where there is an abundance of receptor sites.

Females, in addition to their naturally produced estrogens, may be exposed to synthetic analogs through birth control pills, and then later through hormone replacement therapy. Over the years, receptor sites throughout the body, continually bombarded with these pseudo-estrogens, can go out of whack. These chemicals can become carcinogenic resulting in precancerous tumors.

**Q:** *In Europe, natural products are used much more extensively than they are here in the United States. Why is that so?*

**A:** The governments over there have been paying for medical treatment for their people for so long that they continue to use what is the most effective. Many times this is the natural remedy which has been around forever. This may also be the most inexpensive method. So if it works, and it doesn't cost a lot, why would they change?

In the United States, the pharmaceutical companies have been so aggressive in their marketing, older natural remedies have slowly been phased out. Physicians receive samples to give out freely, and "everyone loves something for nothing." If the drug worked, the doctor wrote a prescription for it. But, many new drugs do not work as safely, effectively or as inexpensively as natural remedies. If there are numerous side effects that go along with it, and you end up having to take something else to counter those side effects, it may not be working all that well after all. Many drugs are developed to treat symptoms rather than the cause of the symptoms. People liked them at first because they felt better right away - but, because the cause was never corrected, the symptoms may continue, thus the individual continues to use the drug. This creates quite a market for the pharmaceutical industry.

Natural remedies are extremely valuable. With the technology that we have today we can now identify the pharmacological constituents in natural products to explain why they work. Don't forget that many of the drugs on the market today originated as natural remedies.

**Q:** *How much supplemental DHEA is recommended?*
**A:** As part of an overall antiaging and disease preven-

tion program, the goal is to create DHEA levels in the body which were naturally occurring when you were in your peak around age 20 or 25. While controversy continues over the proper dosage, starting at small doses of DHEA is recommended: about 5-25 mg daily.

Many physicians prescribe 50 mg daily to women over the age of 60, and 100 mg daily for men over the age of 60. DHEA doses of 500 mg per day may be too high, possibly harming the liver and adrenal glands, and may cause side effects such as acne and unwanted hair growth in women.

Larger therapeutic doses are given to patients with cancer, AIDS, and other serious conditions. High doses may create stress on the liver and adrenals and precautions should be taken. Antioxidants and other nutritional substances should be utilized to help counter possible adverse effects.

Some human studies have used dosages as high as 1,500 mg daily. I would strongly advise against this as the long term effects of taking this much are not known. Therapeutic doses must be under the close supervision of a physician.

The younger a person is the smaller the dosage of DHEA will be needed compared to someone who is older when adrenal output declines further.

It is important to be "in tune" with your body so that you can identify this. Remember DHEA, called the "mother hormone," seems to know what hormones to convert to and where go.

# Appendix I

# Forever Young by Burkhard Bilger

The best way to delay aging in a mouse is to under feed it. In fact mice raised on the edge of starvation not only live between 35 and 40 percent longer than mice allowed to eat their fill; they are also far less likely to contract cancer or autoimmune diseases. The three men having lunch with me knew that - they had spent years trying to stay young by studying what causes people age - but they clearly preferred to leave some fountains of youth untasted. Strolling hack from an opulent hotel buffet, they carried plates in both hands; salmon in tarragon cream and stir-fried duck, buttered rolls and volcanic salads streaming with dressing. It is possible to delay aging, they seemed to think, without making yourself miserable.

"The thing that I've noticed." William Regelson said, settling into his chair, "is a return of morning erections," the immunologist across the table nodded between mouthfuls. "When I started taking DHEA, the change in my libido was so striking that my wife noticed and I noticed," he said. "It was funny at hell. I mean, I felt like I was twenty years old again."

As we ate, snatches of similar conversations drifted over from other tables. For three days in mid June, the New York Academy of Sciences had been hosting a conference at the hotel, titled "Dehydroepiandrosterone (DHEA) and Aging." DHEA is the most plentiful steroid hormone in the human body - and the most poorly understood. Regelson, a medical oncologist at the Medical College of Virginia and co author of "*The Melatonin Miracle*," calls DHEA the mother steroid, because the body converts it into estrogen and testosterone. But DHEA is best known as a bio-marker for age. From youth through early adulthood, the adrenal gland secretes the hormone in steadily rising quantities, then tapers off production as the body declines. At the age of eighty, people have between 80 and 90 percent less DHEA in their blood than they had at the age of twenty-five. Levels of estrogen, testosterone, melatonin and human growth hormone also rise and fall with age, prompting a now familiar question: If the body deteriorates as hormones decline, what happens if those hormones are replaced?

Ice baths, gold elixirs, naps with young virgins, fostering body lice, injecting mashed dog testicles and holding one's breath; cures for aging are perennially proposed and perennially proved futile. But conferences such as this one, which gathered respected investigators from numerous countries and disciplines, signal a new legitimacy for research on aging and on DHEA. Investigators have gotten their first glimpses into how the hormone works; synthetic analogues are being tested; and human trials have begun to yield promising data. Long overshadowed by estrogen, human growth hormone and melatonin, DHEA has finally entered the limelight at a potential "miracle drug." In June, on the CBS television news magazine *Eye to Eye* a segment on DHEA cut between interviews with conference speakers and clips of old-timers regaining their youth in the movie *Cocoon*. Articles about DHEA soon followed in other media, including *The Washington Post, Science* and *The New York Times.*

Drug hype is a constant of popular culture, but stories about DHEA are like trailers for a movie that may never get made. The US Food and Drug Administration has yet to approve DHEA, and few physicians will prescribe it. Thanks to loopholes created by the Dietary Supplement Health and Education Act of 1994, DHEA of varying quality and concentration, synthesized item cytosterol found in Mexican yams, can be bought in health-food stores, mail order houses or compounding pharmacies. But the Drug Enforcement Administration has tentatively defined DHEA as an anabolic steroid; if that definition sticks and the DEA can afford to enforce it, over-the-counter and mail-order sales of the drug will be curtailed. Only FDA approval can rescue the hormone from the grey market. But DHEA has been around too long to be patented and pharmaceutical companies are reluctant to spend hundreds of millions of dollars testing a drug they cannot own. It may be years, in other words before DHEA is widely available-that is, unless clinical tests prove it has disastrous side effects.

For users of antiaging drugs, however, time is understandably of the essence. At the conference, during talks in the hotel ballroom chandelier light gleamed from dozens of balding heads and thick eyeglasses. Professors emeriti clustered around their younger colleagues between sessions, looking for answers, advice and assurance. At the beginning of his talk, the biochemist Arthur G. Schwartz of the Temple University School of Medicine summarized findings that showed DHEA can cause liver cancer in rodents. "I could pick out the people in the audience on DHEA by the way their faces fell." he said afterward, "I would say 25 percent were taking it."

Physicians have a long tradition of testing drugs on themselves. Jonas Salk injected himself and his entire family with the polio vaccine before making it public. But some of the people taking DHEA are also prescribing it, and some have a fundamental problem with the way new drugs are regulated The elderly are as imperiled as AIDS patients are, they say, and should be given similar freedoms to experiment with new drugs. Baby boomers, stumbling through middle age by the millions, are turning toward New Age cures and Chinese medicines. Why not let them restore depleted hormones instead? Why wait for multi-million dollar tests to confirm common sense? This may not be how science works," one DHEA investigator told me. "But it's the way that real life works."

John E. Nestler, one of the conference organizers, has tested his own DHEA level and found it to be below normal for his age. His research has shown that high doses of DHEA can lower the amount of "bad" cholesterol in a person's blood. Yet he will not emulate his DHEA-taking colleagues. "I think that they are really jumping the gun," he says. "People said human growth hormone was great stuff at first too, but now we are seeing significant side effects- bloating, carpal tunnel syndrome. The same thing could happen with DHEA."

At our lunch, digging into a slice of white chocolate mousse, Regelson acknowledged Nestlers' position with a tight shrug. Although the two men are friends and colleagues at the Medical College of Virginia, they have become spokesmen for opposite camps in the DHEA debate. "I respect John Nestler," Regelson said, stifling his exasperation for just a beat. "He's a top-flight scientist. But the guy is forty-two years old! I mean, the guy has just started a family; he is just getting his full professorship; he can afford to be conservative, I'll be seventy on July 12. It's like somebody out there has a contract out to kill me. I don't want to wait twenty or thirty years. I want it now."

Regelson is an old hand at rabble-rousing for research on aging. At the conference, striding up to microphones in suspenders and rolled shirt sleeves, he looked more like a union organizer, a leader of Whobblies than the distinguished oncologist he is. He spoke in a fluid, mesmerizing basso, prodding the audience between explanations "Okay?... Are you with me?... Okay?" His voice growing more emphatic as his arguments piled up. Regelson has a face that vaguely resembles Art Buchwald's, though with swarthier skin, add a body that moves with the heavy-set agility of a badger. But his most striking trait arises from a combination of features: He looks twenty years younger than his age.

DHEA first drew Regelson's attention in 1980. By then, studies in Europe have shown that DHEA could help solve gout, psoriasis and congestive heart problems. More important, Arthur Schwartz had found that DHEA when given to mice, inhibited breast cancer as well as a host of cancers caused by chemical agents. For Regelson, however, the most convincing evidence was the least scientifically conclusive. "In 1982," he remembers, "my mother-in law had a midthigh amputation and became markedly weak, depressed, senile as a post. Here she was living in my house, essentially a vegetable. I threw everything at her except the kitchen sink. It wasn't a study; it was an act of desperation. But lo and behold, when I gave her DHEA she became a normal human being again." Regelson's wife has been taking DHEA ever since he started taking it five years ago.

At first Regelson seemed well placed to promote DHEA. Just as he was gathering information on the hormone, he and Senator Alan M. Cranston were organizing the Fund for Integrative Biomedical Research (FIBER). "The whole concept at FIBER was to look at aging as a syndrome rather than as a random collection of degenerative diseases," he says. I think of the body as a clock, and that clock can be manipulated." Melatonin, Regelson now

219

believes, can actually reset the clock and extend life, DHEA keeps the body disease free and energetic by restoring levels of the two hormones to their youthful peaks, people may be able to add up to thirty healthy years to their lives.

As scientific director of FIBER, Regelson tried for five years to stir up interest in DHEA. He gave away seed money, organized conferences, wrote grant proposals and lobbied The National Institute on Aging to start a DHEA study- all with little success. The medical establishment still dismissed antiaging drugs as high-tech snake oil. Stymied, Regelson wandered elsewhere in the antiaging community, becoming a mentor and provocateur to other DHEA investigators, connecting the dots between data in disparate studies. Ironically, only one year after FIBER folded, a single study triggered the groundswell he had hoped for.

In 1986 Elizabeth Barrett-Connor, an epidemiologist at the University of California, San Diego, reported that among 143 middle-aged and elderly men who had been followed for twelve years, the ones with high DHEA sulfate levels in their blood suffered half as many cases of heart disease as the men with low DHEA levels, "The results were so incredible that I didn't believe them at first," Barrett-Connor says. "So I went back and pulled ninety-nine more blood samples. They showed the same thing." Women in the study who had high DHEA sulfate levels had a slightly higher risk of heart disease, but that bit of bad news was overshadowed by the apparent good news for men.

**The best news of all, however, was reserved for mice.** The flurry of small-scale DHEA studies prompted by Barrett-Connor's findings most involved laboratory mice, which benefited from doses of DHEA in a dizzying variety of ways. DHEA reversed diabetes and inhibited lung cancer, breast cancer and skin cancer. It helped mice lose weight by raising their metabolism and decreasing their appetites; it restored their memory (by encouraging neurite formation in the brain) and relieved stress.

Photographic slides of DHEA successes were much in evidence at the Academy conference. Mice with skin cancer next to mice with perfect skin; old mice with their hair falling out next to mice, just as old, with glistening fur. When the speakers discussed the effects of DHEA on humans, they turned cautious, equivocal. But when they talked about its effects on mice, they had few doubts.

"If rodents don't have this hormone naturally they probably should," says Raymond A. Daynes, an immunologist at the University of Utah School of Medicine. With a high, domed forehead and small eyes that glint behind round glasses, Daynes seems to relish the role of medical master- mind, speaking with clipped, programmatic precision, as if punching hits of information directly into one's brain. For the past six years, he has studied how DHEA-S (the sulfated form of DHEA) affects the mouse immune system, formulating an elegant model of how mice physically deteriorate with age-and how DHEA keeps them from doing so.

Very old mice, like very old people, have immune systems so weak that vaccinations do them little good. But when Daynes gave his mice DHEA-S, their immune systems were suddenly rejuvenated. "It was a clear, 100 percent change," he says. "Now their immune system worked and before it didn't." At the same time, other signs of old age began to fall away. "They were gaining weight instead of losing it; their vitality was greater; we were seeing dramatic alterations in a variety of systems," Daynes says. "Even with quite low levels of DHEA-S, mouse immune systems aged backward for a year. And the mice given DHEA-S invariably outlived mice that were not given the hormone. "After two years, we sometimes had only five out of twenty control animals left," Daynes says. "But nearly all ten of the mice on DHEA-S were still alive."

Daynes began to think that DHEA-S was fixing some mechanism in mice, some faulty part that normally led to a breakdown. "That's when the light bulbs went off," he says. In 1993 his research group had discovered a "leaky faucet": In very old mice the immune system was secreting the cytokine interleukin-6 (IL-6) for no apparent reason. A quick glance at the medical literature showed that many of the problems associated with old age-including many cancers - could be caused by excess quantities of IL-6. Daynes set out to learn how DHEA-S affected excess IL-6 production. "It was dramatic," he says. "Within twenty-four hours of providing the supplement, we no longer had the leaky faucet." His group has since discovered two other hormonal leaks implicated in a host of physical ailments. DHEA-S shuts off both leaks.

**But will it do so in people?** The question murmured through the crowd during every presentation at the conference. DHEA may work wonders in mice, but mice have little of the hormone in their bodies, and they therefore may respond to it differently from the way people do. Many drugs cure cancer in mice for instance, but few cure cancer in humans.

In some clinical trials moderate doses of DHEA and DHEA-S have benefited people: elderly human subjects on DHEA-S were more responsive to influenza vaccines than they were without it; people with lupus (an autoimmune disease) found that DHEA relieves some of their symptoms; aging men and women after taking DHEA in year-long double-blind trial, felt better, slept better and had less soreness in their joints. But the most dramatic effects-the increases in life span that have physicians popping DHEA and hinting at a fountain of youth-have yet to be seen in people, "I'd like to think that I'm not solely building a better mousetrap," Daynes says. But DHEA studies may literally take a lifetime to erase or confirm his hopes.

"Every five years a new wonder drug comes along," Barrett-Connor says. "Well, I don't think DHEA is the wonder drug the people at the meeting seemed to think it is. Nine years after resurrecting DHEA with her study on heart disease, Barrett-Connor is in the ironic position of wanting to rebury it. In a larger follow-up study, she noted that high DHEA levels lowered the risk of heart disease in men by only 20 percent- in line with what several other studies have shown. "Maybe it's good that my new results may help dampen the enthusiasm," she says. "I was astounded that there were physicians out there giving this drug to thousands of people in the absence of any studies about what it does."

If the benefits of DHEA have yet to be proved, some of the risks are clear. Because DHEA affects so many parts of the body, taking it may be akin to swallowing a handful of unmarked pills. Investigators are not sure whether the hormone affects the body directly or by regulating other hormones or by turning into androgens and estrogens-which have problems of their own. To achieve some of the effects observed in mice, people may have to take "super-pharmacological" doses, which have been shown to cause acne and hair growth in women. "When you take it as a pill, the first place it goes is to your liver." Barrett-Connor points out. "Things happen in the liver. Enzymes change it's character, destroy it and do other things we're not aware of." The livers in mice on DHEA enlarge and change color from pink to mahogany. When sixteen rats were fed DHEA for as long as eighty-four weeks in a study at Northwestern University Medical School, fourteen developed liver cancer.

"Anyone who is intimidated by that liver-damage story is an idiot." Regelson says. Why should the body go haywire when it is given as much DHEA as it once naturally produced? According to Regelson, patients taking super-pharmacological doses to fight cancer or AIDS have suffered no liver damage so far. And even if they had, they might be willing to take the risk. As an oncologist who regularly treats advanced cancers, Regelson is used to doling out potentially lethal remedies in experimental trials. He simply asks patients to sign a release acknowledging the dangers of taking an unapproved drug. But most physicians worry that a release is no guarantee against a lawsuit where unapproved drugs are concerned, "I have an eighty-seven-year old friend with chronic heart failure. I want to put him on DHEA but his doctor is too hidebound." Regelson says, "You have a patient who is dying, saying, 'Doctor, please help me.' Some guys wait for a drug to be approved, I won't."

A federal program should be established to identify unpatentable drugs such as DHEA, Regelson believes, offering patent-like protection to drug companies willing to test and develop them. Better still, aging should be considered a life-threatening disease, and antiaging drugs should be put on a fast track for FDA approval, with less-demanding criteria. "Everybody wants a safe society, but you have to see this in terms of a war. You are going to have casualties," he says, "If man were mouse, we would have found the cure for cancer fifty years ago."

Intentionally or not, Regelson's slogans echo the alarms shouted by people even more haunted by their mortality than those who take DHEA: AIDS activists. In the years since the virus appeared they have catalyzed changes in the drug-approval process as complaints from physicians such as Regelson never could. The FDA, criticized in the early 1980s for its sluggish drug trials, has tried to accommodate victims of the virus both by putting new anti-AIDS drugs on a fast track and by looking the other way when unapproved drugs were sold and used on the street.

In the advanced stages of AIDS, patients have next to no DHEA left in their bodies. Restoring the hormone at that point seems to do little good (although in vitro, the hormone inhibits infection of the cells by the virus), but many people who are HIV positive take DHEA to strengthen their immune systems, relieve fatigue and build muscle before the disease takes it away. On the Internet "threads" of DHEA queries and responses stretch back for years. 'The results in my case look hopeful so far," one comment from 1993 reads. "But I think a few more months are necessary before I'd conclude it's the DHEA." The writer has since died, leaving no real evidence whether the hormone delayed or accelerated his condition.

Spencer Cox has a hard time getting too excited about DHEA. As the chair of the antiviral committee of the Treatment Action Group in New York City, he has spent seven years at the epicenter of drug hype. "There comes a point, where you have seen the cure coming down the pipeline over and over again," he says. "And there have been some scares-some bad scares." In 1993, when the drug fialuridine was being tested as a treatment for chronic hepatitis (commonly suffered by patients with AIDS), it seemed relatively safe at first. "A few months later, the patients started dropping dead from liver failure." Cox remembers. "The take-home message was new drugs can be dangerous."

The FDA built its procedural bulwark to defend consumers after similar disasters in the 1930s and 1960s. Results from small-scale tests are not always reliable, experience has shown.

Physicians can consciously or unconsciously pick patients who will respond particularly well to a new drug; or they may conclude that a drug cures a broad array of conditions when it affects only a single symptom. Chastened by their experiences with drugs such as fialuridine, some AIDS activists have reversed their earlier appeals. urging the FDA to test new drugs more thoroughly. "If (a cure) comes along, it will be easy to detect, and we can drop all the rules," Cox says, "In the meantime, we are not dealing with therapeutic effects that are that big."

In medicine, as in government, unfortunately, the strictest standard can foster the most furious, potentially self-defeating search for loop-holes. Because DHEA cannot be patented but must be approved to be widely sold, drug companies are testing  synthetic analogues that lack the natural hormone's side effects. Of course, such analogues could have long-term side effects of their own. And because no company has the time or the money to spend on a fifty-year study to see if a drug extends life, DHEA will likely be approved for specific uses such as treating lupus or in other words, some form of DHEA may be approved and readily available within a few years, but people taking it to stay young will have to continue doing so on the sly, without long-term data to back up their decision.

Antiaging drugs may help people stay healthy or live longer. But no one will know that for sure until most people alive today are dead. Given that paradox, DHEA investigators, like the patients they counsel or inform, have no choice but to rely on mouse studies and inconclusive trials, rumor and anecdote. Raymond Daynes is fifty years old- too young to take DHEA, he says but old enough to watch colleagues such as Regelson with an appreciative eye. "Some of the people at that conference have been taking the hormone for a long time, and they're pretty smart, wily individuals," he says. "They're getting close to eighty years old, but I wouldn't want to play racquetball with them."

This article is reprinted by permission from The New York Academy of Sciences from *The Sciences* (September/October 1995). Individual subscriptions are $21.00 per year. Write to: *The Sciences*, 2 East 63rd Street, New York, New York 10021 or call: 1-800-THE-NYAS.

# GLYCEMIC FOOD VALUES:

*Eating foods with a lower glycemic food value reduces adrenal and endocrine stress.*

| **_Best_** _(low)_ 0-30 | **_OK_** _(med)_ 36-65 | **_Worst_** _(hi)_ 66-100 |
| --- | --- | --- |
| **BREADS:** | | crisp crackers |
| Coarse whole grain wheat or rye | 100% stone ground whole wheat breads or mat-zoh | White bread |
| Pita bread | | Commercial whole wheat breads |
| Cracked or sprouted wholewheat bread | Pumpernickel | Commercial rye bread |
| | 100% whole grain rye | English muffins, bagels, commercial |
| **PASTA/ GRAINS:** | | |
| Pasta (all types) | Brown Rice | Instant, "Quick" or Precooked Grains |
| Barley, Bulgur, Buckwheat Kasha, Couscous | Boiled or Baked Potato | Instant, or one-minute white rice |
| Most Beans Peas Sweet potato / Yam | Lima Beans Whole Corn | |
| **DAIRY:** | | |
| Milk; 1% or skim | 2% Milk | Whole milk, |
| Cottage cheese | Cheese | Ice milk, |
| Buttermilk | Regular and Plain Yogurt | Ice cream |
| low-fat yogurt (plain or w/ fruit) | | Yogurt sweetened with sugar (including low-fat varieties) |
| Yogurt w/ artificial sweetener | | |
| low-fat artificially sweetened desserts | | low-fat frozen desserts with sugar |
| low-fat frozenyogurt w/ artificial sweetener | | low-fat and regular frozen yogurt w/ sugar |

| *Best (low)* 0-30 | *OK (med)* 36-65 | *Worst (hi)* 66-100 |
|---|---|---|

## MEAT/PROTEIN:

| | | |
|---|---|---|
| Shellfish "White" (lowfat) fish, i.e., cod, flounder, trout, tuna in water | Higher fat fish, i.e., salmon, herring | Most cuts of beef, pork, lamb hot dogs (including "lowfat" versions) |
| Egg substitutes (cholesterol-free) | Lean cuts of beef, pork. | Cheese (Regular) |
| Cottage cheese | Low-fat cheese | Luncheon meat |
| Venison | Eggs | Peanut butter, peanuts |
| Skinless chicken, turkey, cornish hen (white meat) | | |

## FRUIT:

| | | |
|---|---|---|
| Most fruit | Natural fruit juices | Pineapple |
| | Kiwi | Raisins/dried fruit |
| | | Watermelon |
| | Mango | Fruit juice (sweetened) |

## VEGETABALES:

| | | |
|---|---|---|
| Almost all vegetables | Beets | Carrots ( high in sugar) Winter Squash (acorn, butternut) |

## SOUP:

| | | |
|---|---|---|
| Most low-fat brands | Most commercial soups (be careful for high fat, high sodium, and starch.) | Powdered or instant soups |

## MISC.:

| | | |
|---|---|---|
| Nuts, almonds, walnuts, etc. | Artificially sweetened deserts | Glucose Sucrose Corn syrup |
| Butter | | Honey Molasses |
| Fructose | | Corn Starch Soft drinks |
| Sugar-free gelatin | | Desserts Candy |

# About The Authors...

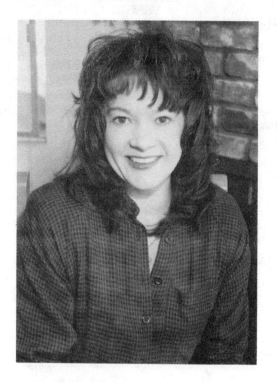

## Beth M. Ley Jacobs

Beth has been a science writer specializing in health and nutrition for 10 years. She wrote her own degree program and graduated in Scientific and Technical Writing from North Dakota State University in 1987 (a combination of Zoology and Journalism). Since then she has written a number of nutrition books including *Castor Oil: It's Healing Properties* (1990), *Dr. John Willard on Catalyst Altered Water* (1990), *Natural Healing Handbook* (1995), *How to Fight Osteoporosis and Win: The Miracle of Microcrystalline Hydroxyapatite (MCHC)* (1996), *The Potato Antioxidant: Alpha Lipoic Acid* (1996) *and Colostrum: Nature's Gift To The Immune System* (1997).

228

She co-authored ***How Did We Get So Fat?*** (1994) with nutritionist Dr. Arnold J. Susser, R.Ph., Ph.D., who has a nutrition counseling practice in Westfield, N.J. (These books are all available through BL Publications.)

Beth makes regular guest radio and television appearances. Look for her on the Inspiration Channel and other Christian radio and television broadcasts. She also lectures nationwide on ***Taking DHEA Responsibly*** to encourage safe, responsible use of DHEA and other hormonal supplements.

Beth is currently working towards her masters degree in nutrition and eventually, plans to obtain her doctorate.

Beth lives in southern California with her husband Randy, and dogs, NaTasha and Cameo. She is dedicated to spreading the health message, regularly attends the gym, eats a vegetarian, lowfat diet and takes anti-aging supplements.

Memberships:
American Academy of Anti-aging
New York Academy of Sciences
Oxygen Society

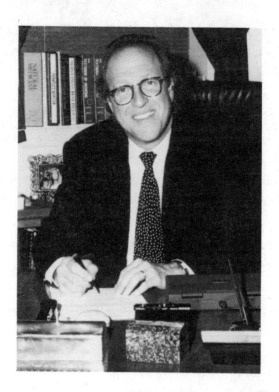

# Richard Ash, M.D.

Dr Richard Ash is a leader in the field of environmental medicine, integrating the best of his Internal Medicine background with the most advanced technology in Alternative Medicine to offer innovative treatments to his patients. This combination can achieve dramatic lasting improvement and has been successful in helping patients who have found conventional methods to be unsuccessful.

Dr Ash bases his practice philosophy on treating the body as a whole. By asserting his beliefs that contemporary medicine has failed because it only treats a patient's symptoms rather than treating the cause of the problem he has become an opinion leader in the field of Alternative Medicine. His new approach to medicine focuses on the body as a working entity where all parts must work in harmony to achieve optimal health. He works to determine and treat underlying causes of an illness and to teach his patients a new way of living in their toxic environment.

Dr. Ash works to educate the public on survival in today's polluted environment through his radio talk show, regular appearances in the media and the publication of targeted articles. His talk show, "In The Doctor's Office." is broadcast each Sunday on 710 AM WOR radio, 5:00 - 7:00 pm, in New York.

Dr. Ash began his collegiate education by receiving a Bachelor of Arts at the University of Cincinnati in 1970. He graduated from the Medical College of Pennsylvania in 1976.

Dr. Ash completed an internship and residency in internal medicine at hospitals affiliated with the Downstate Medical Center from 1976-1979. In 1979 he began his private practice. Dr Ash is licensed by the State of New York in internal medicine.

Dr Ash has become well known for successful alternative treatments and patients travel nationally and internationally to seek his advice. He treats a wide variety of clientele. including celebrities and athletes.

Dr. Ash has made numerous radio and TV appearances, several times on America's Talking with Carol Martin and most recently, on ABC's World News Tonight with Peter Jennings.

Dr. Ash was born in New York City and raised in New Rochelle. He enjoys staying active in golf, tennis and other sports, in addition to his strenuous work schedule. He and his wife love and own several Yorkies.

Dr. Ash believes that his unique approach to medicine will make an impact on the overall quality of optimal health people can achieve and feels that through education, this type of treatment will become model for the rest of the country to follow.

Memberships:
Academy of Environmental Medicine
American Academy of Preventive Medicine
American College of Advancement in Medicine (ACAM)
American Society of Bariatric Physicians
Foundation for Advancements in Innovative Medicine (FAIM)
Great Lakes Association of Clinical Medicine (GLACM)
Medical Society of New York

# BIBLIOGRAPHY

Abbasi, A., Mattson, D.E., et al, " "Hyposmatomedinemia and hypogonadism in hemiplegic men who live in nursing homes." Arch Phys Med Rehabil, 1994 May; 75(5):594-599.

Adains, J.B., Archiblad, K., Seymour-Munn, Cancer Res (4), 1980; 3815-3820.

Adams, J.B., Cancer (40), 1977; 325-332.

Adams, J.B., Wong, M.S.F., J. Endocrinol. (41), 1968; 41-52.

Adams, J.B., Molec. & Cell Endocrinol. (41), 1985; 1-17.

Adinoff B, Martin PR, Eckardt MJ, Linnoila M "Role of DHEA and DHEA-S in Alzheimer's disease" Am J Psychiatry 1993 Sep;150(9):1432-3

Ahluwalia B, Smith D, et al "Ethanol decreases progesterone synthesis in human placental cells: mechanism of ethanol effect" Alcohol 1992 Sep-Oct;9(5):395-401

Aksoy, L.A., Wood, T.C., Weinshilboum, R., "Human liver estrogen sulfotransferase: identification by DNA cloning and expression." Biochem Biophys Res Commun 200(3), 1994 May 16; 1621-1629.

Albrecht, E.D., Henson, M.C., et al "Modulation of adrenocorticotropin-stimulated baboon fetal adrenal dehydroepiandrosterone formation in vitro by estrogen at mid- and late gestation." Endocrinology 126(6), 1990 Jun; 3083-3088.

Ali, S.A., Schoonen, E.J., et al., Gen. Comp Endor. (66), 1987; 415-424.

Alper, M.M., Garner, M.B., Fertil. and Sterility (47), 1987; 255-258.

Amer. J. Publ. Health, 1988; Sept-Oct.

Anapliotou, M.G., Sygrios, K., et al., "Adrenal hyperresponsiveness to ACTH stimulation in women with polycystic ovary syndrome; an adrenarchal type of response." J. Clin. Endocrinol Metab 71(4), 1990 Oct; 900-906.

Anderson, J., "Independence of the effects of cholesterol and degree of saturation of the fat in the diet on serum cholesterol in man.: Am J Clin Nut, 29 (1976); 1884.

Arad, Y., Badimon, J.J., Badimon, L., et al., Arteriosclerosis (9), 1989; 159-166.

Aradhana, Rao., A.R., Kale, R.K., "Diosgenin—a growth stimulator of mammary gland of ovariectomized mouse." Indian J. Exp. Biol. 30(5), 1992 May; 367-370.

Araneo BA; Ryu SY; Barton S; Daynes RA "Dehydroepiandrosterone reduces progressive dermal ischemia caused by thermal injury." J Surg Res 1995 Aug;59(2):250-62

Argtielles, A.E., et al., Endocrine profiles and breast cancer. Lancet, 1973; 1:165-168.

Attanasio, A., Robkamp, R., Bernasconi, S., et al., Ped.Red. (22), 41-44.

Bannister, P., Oakes, J., Sheridan, P., et al., Quart. J. Ned. (63), 1987; 305-313.

Banrett-Connor, E., Rhaw, K.T., Yen, S.S.C., "A prospective study of dehydroepiandrosterone sulfate, mortality, and cardiovascular disease." N Eng J Med, 1986; 315:1519-1524.

Barkan, A., Cassorla, F., Loriaunx, P.L., et al., Obs. Gynecol. (64), 1984; 287-295.

Barnard, J., "Response of non-insulin-dependent diabetic patients to an intensive program of diet and exercise." Diabetes Core 5, 1982; 370.

Barrett-Conor, E., Edelstein, S.L., "A prospective study of dehydroepiandrosterone sulfate and cognitive function in an older population: The Rancho Bernardo Study." J. Am. Geriatr. Soc. 42(4), 1994 Apr.; 420-423.

Barrett-Conor, E., Khaw, K.T., N. Eng. J. Med. (317), 1987; 711.

Barrett-Conor, E., Khaw, K.T., Yen, S.S.C., N. Eng. J. Med. (315), 1986; 1519-1524.

Beaton, G., "Practical population health indicators of health and nutrition." WHO Monograph, 62(1976); 500.

Becchi, M., Aguilera, R., et al., "Gas chromatography/combustion/istoope-ratio mass spectrometry analysis of urinary steroids to detect misuse of testosterone in sport." Rapid Common Mass Spectrum 8(4), 1994 Apr; 304-308.

Becker U "The influence of ethanol and liver disease on sex hormones and hepatic oestrogen receptors in women." Dan Med Bull 1993 Sep;40(4):447-59

Begin, D., Luthy, I.A., Labrie, F., Moled. & Cellular Endocrinol. (5), 1988; 213-219.

Becker U, Gluud C, et al "Menopausal age and sex hormones in postmenopausal women with alcoholic and non-alcoholic liver disease." J Hepatol 1991 Jul;13(1):25-32.

Begchi, N., Brown, T.R., Shieris, B., et al., Endocrinol (109), 1981; 1428-1432.

Behre, H.M., Bohmeyer, J., Nieschlag, E., "Prostate volume in testosterone-treated and untreated hypogonadal men in comparison to age-matched normal controls." Muns Clin Endocrinol, (Oxf) 1994 Mar; 40(3):341-349.

Belanger, B., Belanger, A., Labrie, F., J. Stero Biochem. (32), 1989; 695-698.

Belanger, B., Caron, S., Belanger, A., Dupont, A., "Steroid fatty acid esters in adrenals and plasma:effects of ACTH." Clin Chem 36(12), 1990 Dec; 2042-2046.

Bell H, Raknerud N., et al "Inappropriately low levels of gonadotrophins in amenorrhoeic women with alcoholic and non-alcoholic cirrhosis" Eur J Endocrinol 1995 Apr;132(4):444-9

Ben-David, B., Dikstein, S., Bismuth, B., Sulm, F.G., Proc Soc., Exp. Med. Biol. (125), 1967; 1136-1140.

Bendayn, M., Reddy, J.K., Lab. Invest. (47), 1982; 364-369.

Berger, E.A., Shapiro, L.J., J. Inher. Metab. Dis. (11), 1988; 403-415.

Bernstein, L., "Relationship of hormones use to cancer risk. Exogenous hormones are widely prescribed in the United States, primarily as oral contraceptives and hormone-replacement therapy." Monogr Natl Cancer Inst, 1992; (12):137-147.

Bing, C., Xu, S.E., Zhang, G.D., Wang, W.Y., Ann. Human Biol. (15), 1988; 421-429.

Berkenhager-Gillesse, E.G., et al., "Dehydroepiandrosterone sulphate (DHEA-S) in the oldest old, aged 85 and over." Ann N Y Acad Sci (719), May 31, 1994; 543-552.

Blaver, K.L., et al., Proc. Ain. Soc. Endocrinol. Abs. (25), 1989; 29.

Boccardo, F., Valent, G., Zanardi, S., et al., Cancer Res. (48), 1988; 5860-5863.

Boizel, R., dePeretti, E., Cathiard, A.M., et al., Clin. Endocrinol. (25), 1986; 363-371.

Bodis J, Tinneberg HR, Schwarz H et al "The effect of histamine on progesterone and estradiol secretion of human granulosa cells in serum-free culture." Gynecol Endocrinol 1993 Dec;7(4):235-9

Bolt HM "Interactions between clinically used drugs and oral contraceptives." Environ Health Perspect 1994 Nov;102 Suppl 9:35-8

Bonney, T.C., Scanlow, N.J., Jones, D.L., J. Endocr. (101), 1985; 181-188.

Bosse, I.K., et al., Arch. Derm. Forsch. (243), 1972; 177-187.

Boyer, Et al., Am J of Clin. Nutr, 1988; 48:896-900.

Bradlow, H.L., Gillette, P.N., Gallagher, K.A., J. Exp. Med (130), 1973; 754-763.

Brehm, E., et al., Arch. Clin. Exp. Derm (234), 1969; 117-124.

Brody, S., Carlstrom, K., Largelius, A., et al., Maturias (4), 1982; 113-118.

Browne, E.S., et al., "Dehydroepiandrosterone: Antiglucoconicoid action in mice." Am J Med Sci, 1992; 303:366-371.

Bulbrook, R.D., Hayward, J.L., Spicer, C.C.F., Lancet (2), 1971; 395-398.

Buchanan, J.R., Hospodar, P., et al., J. Clin. End. Metab. (67), 1988; 937-943.

Buffington, C.K., Givens, J.R., Kitbachi, A.E., Clin. Res. (36), 1988; 41.

Buffington, C.K., Givens, J.R., Kitbachi, A.E., "Enhanced adrenocortical activity as a contributing factor to diabetes in hyperandrogenic women." J. Endocrinol 140(2), 1994 Feb; 297-307.

Calabrese, B.P., Isaacs, E.R., Regelson, W., "Dehydroepiandrosterone in multiple sclerosis: positive effects on fatigue syndrome in a non-randomizing study. In the biological role of dehydroepiandrosterone." edited by M. Kalimi and W. Regelson, New York: de Gruyter, 1990; 95-100.

Carlstrom, K., Brody, S., Lunell, N.O., Maturitas (10), 1988; 297-306.

Carlstrom, K., Stege, R., "Adrenocortical function in prostatic cancer patients: effects of orchidectomy or different modes of estrogen treatment on basalsteroid levels and on the response to exogenous adrenocorticotropic hormone." Urol. Int. 45(3), 1990; 160-163.

Carmina, E., Lobo, R.A., "Pituitary-adrenal responses to ovine corticotropin-releasing factor in polycystic ovary syndrome and other hyperandrogenic patients." Gynecol Endocrinol 4(4), 1990 Dec; 225-232.

Casazza, J.P., Schaeffer, W.T., Veech, R.L., Nutr. (116), 1986; 304-310.

Casey, M.L., Shackleton, C.H.K., et al. J. Steroid Biochem. (30), 1988; 1-6.

Castagnetti, L., "Short report on the 5th symposium on the analysis of steroids." Steroids 59(1), 1994 Jan; 55-56.

Cayen, M.N., Dvornick, D., "Effect of diosgenin on lipid metabolism in rats." J. Lipid Res. 20(2), 1979 Feb; 162-167.

Chakravorty, J., Br. J. Dermatol. (83), 1970; 477-481.

Chasalow, F.I., Blethen, S.L., Bradlow, H.L., Steroids. (52); 205-215.

Chasalow, F.I., Blethen, Jobash, J.G., Am. J. Med. Genetics. (28), 1987; 857-864.

Cisternino, M., "Transdermal estradiol substitution therapy for the induction of puberty in female hypogonadism." J Endocrinol Invest, 1991 Jun; 14 (6):481-488.

Cleary, M.P., Shepherd, P., Jenits, B., "Effect of dehydroepiandrosterone on growth in lean and obese Zucker rats." J Nutr, 1984; 114:1242-1251.

Clerici, M., Bevilacqua, M., Vago, T., et al., "An immunoendocrinological hypothesis of HIV infection." Lancet 343(8912), June 18, 1994; 1552-1553.

Coleman, D.L., Laiter, E.H.., Applerweig, N., "Therapeutic effects of dehydroepiandrosterone metabolities in diabetes mutant mice." Endocrinology, 1984; 115, 239-243.

Colgan, M., Fielde, S., Colgan, L.A., "Micronutrient status of endurance athletes affects hematology and performance." J. Appi. Nutr. Vol (43), No. 1, 1991; 17-36.

Conget, J.I., Halperin, I., Ferrer, J., Gonzalez, Clemente, J.M., Martinez, Osaba, M.J., Vilardell, E., "Evaluation of clinical and hormonal effects in hirsute women treated with keto conazole." J. Endocrinol Invest. 13(11), 1990 Dec; 867-870.

Corpechot, C., LeClerc, P., Baulieu, E.E., Brazeau, P., (45), 1985; 229-234.

Crilly, R.G., Marshall, D.H., Nordin, B.E.C., "Metabolic effects of corticosteroid therapy in post-menopausal women." J Steroid Biochem, 1979; 11:429-433.

Crudo, D.F., Proc. Am. Soc. Endocrinol. Abs. (1455), 1989; 386.

Culig, Z., Hobisch, A., et al., "Mutant androgen receptor detected in an advanced-stage prostatic carcinoma as activated by adrenal androgens and progesterone." J. Immunol 152(7), 1994 Apr 1; 3417-3426.

Cummings., D.C., "Androgenesit and androdynamics in normal women." Cleve. Clin. J. Med. 57(2), 1990 Mar-Apr; 161-166.

Cummings, D.C., Rebar, R.W., Hopper, B.R., Yen, S.S., J. Clin. Endocrinol. Metab. (54), 1982; 1069-1071.

David S., Nathaniel, E.J.H., Exp. Neurol., 1981; 243-253.

Davis, P.J., Davis, F.B., Blas, S.D., Life Sci. (30), 1982; 675-682.

de Lignieres, B., "Transdermal dihydrotestosterone treatment of 'andropause'." Ann Med, 1993 Jun; 25(3):235-241.

Denckla, W.D., Mech. Aging & Develop. (6), 1977; 143-152.

Dennenbaum, R., Hoffman, G., Oertel, G.W., Horm Metab. Res. (4), 1972; 383-385.

DePeretti, G., Forest, N.G., J. Clin. Endocr. Metab (47), 1978; 572-577.

Derogatis, L.R., Rose, L.I., Shulman, L.H., et al., "Serum androgens and psychopathology in hirsute women." J Psychosm Obstet Gynaecol 14(4), 1993 Dec; 12469-4282.

Deshpande, N., Yates, J., J. Endocrinol. (59), 1971; 35.

Deslypere, J.P., DeBiscop, G., Vermeulen, A., Clin. Endocrinol. (18), 1983; 25-30.

Deuster, P.A., et al., "Nutritional intakes and status of highly trained amenorrheic and cnmenorrheic women runners." Fertil. Steril. (46), 1986; 636.

Dettling M, Heinz A, et al "Dopaminergic responsivity in alcoholism: trait, state, or residual marker?" Am J Psychiatry 1995 Sep;152(9):1317-21

Deutsch, S., Benjamin, F., Seltzer, V., et al., J. Gyinecol. Obstet. (25), 1987; 217-222.Devesa, J., Perez-Fernandez, R., et al., Horm. Metabol. Res. (20), 1988; 57-60.

Devogelaer, J.P., Crabbe, J., DeDeuxchaisnes, C.N., "Bone mineral density in Addison's disease: Evidence for an effect of adrenal adrogens on bone mass." Br Med J, 1987; 294:798-800.

Diamond, P., Brisson, G.R., et al., Eur. J. Appl. Physol. (58), 1989; 699-770.

DiBlasio, A.M., et al., "Maintenance of cell proliferation and steroidogenesis in cultured human fetal adrenal cells chronically exposed to adrenocorticotropic hormone: rationalization of in vitro and in vivo findings." Biol Reprod 42(4), 1990 Apr; 683-691.

Dogliotti. L., et al., Br. J. Cancer Res (22), 1986; 1301-1307.

Doldin, B., "Estrogen excretion patterns and plasma levels in vegetarian and omnivorous women." N Engl J. Med 307, 1982; 1:1542.

Drocker, W.D., Blumberg, J.M., et al., "Biologic activity of dehydroepiandrosterone sulfate in man." Journal of Clinical Encodrinology, 1972; 35, 48-50.

Drucker, W.D., Bull. N.Y. Acad. Med (53), 347-357.

Duffy, P.H., Fevers, R.J., Leakey, J.A., et al., Mech. Age Develop. (48), 1989; 117-133.

Dyerberg, J., "Haemostatic function and platelet polyunsaturated fatty acids in Eskimos." Lancet 2, 1979; 433.

Ebeling, P., Koivisto, V.A., "Physiological importance of dehydroepiandrosterone." Eng J Clin Endocrinol Metab 78(6), 1994 Jun; 15-20.

Ehrmann, D.A., Rosenfield, R.L., "Hirsutism ƒbeyond the steroidogenic block." N. Engl. J. Med. 323(13), 1990 Sept 27; 909-911.

Eich, D.M., Johnson, D.E., Nestler, J.E., Clin. Res. In Press., 1990;

Elliot, D.L., et al., Am. J. Clin. Nutr (49), 1989; 93.

Engelken, S.F., Eaton, R.P., Atherosclerosis, 1981; 177-188.

Enzi, G., et al., eds. Obesity: Pathogenesis and Treatment, New York: Academic Press, 1981.

Erenus, M., et al., "Comparison of the efficacy of spironolactone versus flutamide in the treatment of hirstuism." Gynecol Endocrinol 7(4), 1994 Dec; 273-277.

Evans, W.S., Schiebinger, R.J., Kaiser, D.L., et al., Endocrinol. (101), 1982; 235-241.

Evers, C.L., J. Amer. Dietetic Assoc. (87), 1987; 66.

Faasati, P., Fassati, M., et al., "Treatment of stabilized liver cirrhosis by dedroepiandisterone." Agressologia 14(4), 1973; 259-268.

Faber, M., Spinnler-Benade, A.J., "Mineral and vitamin intake in field athletes (Discuss-Hammer, Havelin-Throwers and Shotputers)." Int. J. Sports Med. Vol(12), No. 3, 1991; 324-327.

Falus, A., et al., "Hormonal regulations of complement biosynthesis in human cell linesƒI. Androgens and gamma-interferon stimulate the biosynthesis and gene expression of C1 inhibitor in human cell lines U937 and HepG2." Mol. Immunol. 27(2), 1990 Feb; 191-195.

Faredin, I., Toth, I., Fazekas, A.G., J. Endocr. (41), 1968; 295-296.

Farinati F, De Maria Net al "Hepatocellular carcinoma in alcoholic cirrhosis: is sex hormone imbalance a pathogenetic factor?" Eur J Gastroenterol Hepatol 1995 Feb;7(2):145-50.

Farmer, R.W., Harrington, C.A., Brain Res. (66), 1974; 552-556.

Fava, M., Rosenbaum, J.F., MacLaughlin, R.A., et al., Psych. Res. (28), 1988; 345-350.

Fava, M., Littman, Halperin, P., Intl. J. Psychiatry in Med. (17), 1987; 289-307.

Fava, M., Halperin, P., Littman, A., et al., Neuro-Endocrinology Letters. (9), 1987; 189.

Fertility and Sterility, Vol 26, No. 1, January 1975.

Ferraccioli G; Guerra P; Rizzi V; Bartoli E "Cyclosporin A increases somatomedin C insulin-like growth factor I levels in chronic rheumatic diseases." J Rheumatol 1995 Jun;22(6):1060-4

Fishere, M.C., LaChance, P.A., "Nutrition evaluation of published weight reducing diets." J. Amer. Dietet Assoc. (85), 1985; 450-454.

Flood, J.F., Roberts, E., Brain Res., 1988; (488), 178-181.

Forest, M.G., dePeretti, E., David, N., Sempe, N., Annales d'Endocrinol. (Paris)(43), 1982; 465-495.

Forrest, A.P.M., Proc. R. Soc. Med. (64), 1971; 509-516.

Fregly, N.J., Threatte, R.M., Life Sci. (30), 1982; 58-59.

Froosmer, D., "Changing age of the Menopause." Br Med J 2, 1964; 349.

Fukieda, K., Faiman, C., et al., J. Clin. Endocrinol. Metab. (53), 1981; 690-693.

Furman, R.H., Howard, R.P., Metabolism. (11), 1962; 93.

Gaby, A., Preventing and Reversing Osteoporosis, Prima Publishing, 1994; 157-172.

Gaillard, R.C., Riondel, A.M., Ling, N., Muller, A.F., Life Sci. (43), 1988; 1935-1944.

Garcea, R., Daino, L., Frassetio, S., et al., Carcinogenesis (9), 1988; 931-938.

Gavaler JS "Alcohol effects on hormone levels in normal postmenopausal women and in postmenopausal women with alcohol-induced cirrhosis." Recent Dev Alcohol 1995;12:199-208

Gavaler JS., Van Thiel DH., et al "Hormonal status of postmenopausal women with alcohol-induced cirrhosis: further findings and a review of the literature." Hepatology 1992 Aug;16(2):312-9.

Gilad, S., Chayen, R., Tordjman, K., et al., "Assessment of 5 alpha-reductase activity in hirsute women: comparison of serum androstanediol glucuronide with urinary androsterone and aeticholanolone excretion." Clin. Endocrinol (Oxf) 40(4), 1994 Apr; 459-464.

Givens, J.R., Ainderson, R.N., et al., J. Clin. Endocrinol. Metab. (40), 988-1000.

Gladstar, R., "Herbal healing for women." Simon and Schuster, New York, NY, 1993; 183-258.

Gomathi C., Balasubramanian K., et al "Effect of chronic alcoholism on semen—studies on lipid profiles." Int J Androl 1993 Jun;16(3):175-81.

Gonzalez, C., Montoya, E., Jolin, T., Gonzalez, N., Endocrinol. (107), 1982; 2099=3004.

Gordon, G., Linib, D., New England Journal of Medicine, 1986; 315, 1519-1522.

Gordon, G., Bush, D., Weisman, H., "Reduction of atherosclerosis by administration of dehydroepiandrosterone." J. Clin Invest., Department of Medicine, Johns Hopkins Medical Institutions, 1988 Aug; 82(2):712-720.

Gordon, G.B., Shantz, L.M., Talalay, P., "In hormones, thermogenesis and obesity." (H.A. Lardy and B. Stratman, eds.). Elsevier, New York, 1989; 339-354.

"Grapefruit juice interactions with drugs." Med Lett Drugs Ther 1995 Aug 18; 37(955): 73-74

Griffith, H., Winter, M.D., "Complete guide to prescription and non-prescription drugs." The Body Pres, Los Angeles, CA, 1988.

Grunwald, K., Rabe, T., Urbancsek, J., Runnebaum, B., Vecsei, P., "Normal values for a short-time ACTA intravenous and intramuscular stimulation test in women in the reproductive age." Gynecol Endocrinol 4(4), 1990 Dec; 287-306.

Guarneri, P., Guameri, R., Cascio, C., Pavasant, P., et al "Neurosteroidogenesis in rat retinas." Mol Cell Endocrinol 99(2), 1994 Mar; 145-151.

Haffa AL; MacEwen EG; Kurzman ID; Kemnitz JW "Hypocholesterolemic effect of exogenous dehydroepiandrosterone administration in the rhesus monkey." In Vivo 1994 Nov-Dec;8(6):993-997.

Haffner, S.M., Valdez, R.A., Mykkanen, L., Stern, M.P., Katz, M.S., "Decreased testosterone and dehydroepiandrosterone sulfate concentrations are associated with increased insulin and glucose concentrations in nondiabetic men." Metabolism, 1994 May; 43(5):599-603.

Hakkinen, K., Pakarinen, A., "Serum hormones and strength development during strength training in middle-aged and elderly males and females." Finland, Acta Physiol Scand, 1994 Feb; 150(2):211-219.

Hardwick, A.J., Linton, E.A., Rothwell, N.J., Enocrinol. (124), 1684-1688.

Harrison, D.E., Archer, J.R., Astle, C.M., J. Immnol. (129), 1982; 2673-2678.

Harvey, W., Grahme, R., Panay, G.S., Ann. Rheum. Dic. (32), 1971; 272-278.

Hastings, L.A., Pashko, L.L., Lenbart, M.L., Schwartz, A.G., Carcinogenesis (9), 1988; 1099-1102.

Heffner, J.E., Milain, M., Ain. J. Respir. Cell Mol. Biol. (2), 1990; 257-261.

Heinonen, P.K., Koivlial, T., Pystynen, P., Gynecol. Obstet. Invest. (23), 1987; 271-274.

Henderson E; Yang JY; Schwartz A "Dehydroepiandrosterone (DHEA) and synthetic DHEA analogs are modest inhibitors of HIV-1 IIIB replication. AIDS Res Hum Retroviruses 1992 May;8(5):625-31

Herbert, L., et al., J. Lipid Res. (15), 1974; 580.

Herecz, P., Ungar, L., Siklos, P., Farguhanson, R.G., Europ. J Obs. & Gyn. & Repor. Biol. (29), 1988; 1-5.

Higuchi, K., et al., Horm. Metab. Res. (17), 1985; 451-453.

Hill, M., "Gut bacteria and aetiology for cancer of the breast." Loncet 2, 1971; 472.

Hill, P., "Plasma hormones and lipids in men at different risk for coronary heart disease." Am J. Clin Nutr 22, 1980; 1010.

Hill, P., "Diet and porlactin Release." Lancet 2, 1976; 806.

Hill P., "Diet and endocrine control." Cancer 39, 1977; 1820.

Hoffman, G., Modsches, B., Dohler, U., Rach. Derm Forsch. (243), 1972; 18-30.

Hollo, I., et al., "Osteopenia" Ann Intern Med, 1977; 86: 637.

Holzman, H., Krapp, R., Morsches, B., et al., Aerptliche Forsch. (25), 1971; 345-353.

Holzman, H., Morsches, B., et al., Arch. Derm. Forsch. (247), 1973; 23-28.

Huggins, C., Mainzer, K., J. Exp. Med (105), 1957; 485-499.

Huot, R.I., Shain, S.A., J. Steroid Biochem (29), 1988; 617-621.

Hursting SD; Perkins SN; Haines DC; Ward JM; Phang JM "Chemoprevention of spontaneous tumorigenesis in p53-knockout mice." Cancer Res 1995 Sep 15;55(18):3949-53

Ingle, J.N., N. Eng. J. Med. (322), 1990; 329-331.

Inano H; Ishii-Ohba H; Suzuki K; et al "Chemoprevention by dietary dehydroepiandrosterone against promotion/progression phase of radiation-induced mammary tumorigenesis in rats." J Steroid Biochem Mol Biol 1995 Jul;54(1-2):47-53

Ito, D., Katsufumi, S., Snao, H., et al., Chem. Pharm. Bull. 34, 1986; 2118-2125.

Ito, D., "Without estrogen, natural remedies for menopause and beyond." Carol Southern Books, New York, NY, 1994; 114, 202, 205.

Iwasaki, M., Darden, T.A., Parker, C.E., Tomer, K.B., Pedersen, L.G., Negishi, M., "Inherent versatility of P450 oxygenase. Conferring dehydroepiandrosterone bydroxylase activity to P-450 2a-4 by a single amino acid mutation at position 117." Breast Cancer Res Treat (3), 1990 Oct, 16; 261-272.

Iwashita, M., Mimuro, T., Watanabe, M., Setoyama, T., Matsuo, A., Adachi, T., Takeda, Y., Sakamoto, S., "Plasma levels of insulin-like growth factor-I and its binding protein in polycystic ovary syndrome." Horm. Res. 33 Suppl. 2, 1990; 21-26.

Jackson, J.A., Fachine, J.K.D., Mellinger, R.C., J. Endocrinol. Invest (12), 1989; 269-272.

Jacobson, M.A., et al. "Decreased derum dehydroepiandrosterone is associated with an increased progression of human immunodeficien' virus infectin in men with CD4 cell counts of 200-499." J Infect Disease, 1991; 164:864-868.

Jesse, R. et al. "DHEA Inhibits Human Platelet Aggregation in Vitro and in Vivo." Annals New York Academy of Sciences, 774, 1995 281-290.

Jimenez J, Osuna C, et al "Effect of chronic ethanol administration on the rat pineal N-acetyltransferase and thyroxine type II 5'-deiodinase activities." Biosci Rep 1993 Apr;13(2):91-8

Jolesz, M., Faredin, I., Toth, I., Acta Med. Hung. 22, 1966; 49-52.

Jones, D.L., James, V.H.T., J. Steroid Biochem 26, 1987; 151-159.

Josephs, J.A., Roth, G.S., Whitaker, J.R., "In interention in the aging process." Part 2, (W. Regelson and N. Sinex, eds.) Alan R. Liss, New York, 1983; 187-202.

Juarez-Oropeza, M.A., Diaz-Zagoya, J.C., Rabinowitz, J.L., "In vivo and in vitro studies of hypocholesterolemic effects of diosgenin in rats." Int. J. Biochem. 19(8), 1987; 679-683.

Kgawa, Y. "Impact of westernization of the nutrition of Japanese: Changes in physique, cancer, longevity, and centenarians.: Prev Med 7, 1978; 205.

Kalimi, M., Regelson, W., Biochem. Biophys. Res. Commun. (156), 1988; 22-29.

Kasic, J.M., et al., Cleve Clin. Q. 50, 1983; 11-22.

Kask, E., Aingiology. (10), 1959; 358-68.

Katz, S.H., Hediger, N.L., et al., Human Biol. (57), 1985; 401-413.

Keizer, H.A., Van Soest, O.P., Kuipers, H., Beckers, E., Med. Sci. in Sports and Exercise (16), 1984; 118-119.

Keller, P.J., Lyskienicz, A., Huch, R., Gynecol. Obstet. Invest. (15), 1983; 365-371.

Kern, P.A., et al., "The effects of weight loss on the activity and expression of adipose tissue lipoprotein lipase in very obese humans." N. engi. J. Med. (322), 1990; 1053.

Keys, A., "Serum cholesterol response to changes in dietary lipids." Am J Clin Nut 19, 1966; 175.

Khalil, M.W., Strutt, B., Vachon, D., et al., "Effects of dexamethasone and cytochrome P450 inhibitors on the formation of 7 alpha-hydroxydehdroepiandros-terone by human adipose stromal cells." J. Steroid Biochem. Mol. Biol. 48 (5-6), 1994 Apr; 545-552.

Khorram, O., Yen, S.S., et al. "Activation of immune function by DHEA in age-advanced men" J Gerontol A Bio Sci Med Sci. 1997; 52:1-7.

Khoury, M.Y., Barachat, E.C., Pardini, D.P., Vieira, J.G., deLima, G.R., "Serum levels of androstanediol glucuronide, total testosterone, and free testosterone in hirsute women." Atherosclerosis 105(2), 1994 Feb; 191-200.

Kirchner, M., The role of hormones in the dtiology of human breast cancer." Cancer 39, 1977; 2716.

Koo, E., Fehr, K.G., Fehr, T., Fust, G., Klin Woehenschr. (61), 1983; 715-717.

Krieg, M., Nass, R., Tunn, S., "Effects of aging on endogenous level of 5 alpha-dihy-drotestosterone, testosterone, estradiol, and estrone in epithelium and stroma of nor-mal and hyperplastic human prostate." J. Clin. Endocrinol. Metab, 1993 Aug; 77(2):375-38.

Kundu, A.K., Sharma, A.K., "A rapid screening technique for detection of diosgenin through in situcytophotometry." Stain Technol 63(6), 1988 Nov; 369-372.

Kurtz, J.W., Wells, W., J. Biol. Chem. (256), 1981; 10870-10875.

Kurtz, B.R., Givens, J.R., et al., J. Clin. Endocrinol. Metab. (64), 1262-1267.

Kung, N.P., Spaulding, S.W., Roth, J.A., Endocrinol (122), 1195-1200.

Labrie, C., Belanger, A., Labrie, F., Endocrinol. (123), 1980; 1412-1417.

Lacroix, C., Fiet, J., Benais, J.P., et al., J. Steroid Biochem. (28), 1987; 317-375.

LaPlante, C., Branchaud, C., Gates, Goodyear, C., Kipowski, S., J. Clin Endocrinol. Metab. (56), 1983; 761-766.

Lanthier, A., Patwardhan, V.V., J. Steroic Biochem. (28), 1987; 697-701.

Lardy, H., Stratinan, F., "Hormones, thermogenesis, and obesity." Elsevier, New York, 1988; 337-452.

Lardy, H., Ching-Yuan, S., Kneer, N., Wieglus, S., "In thermogenesis & obesity." (H. Lardy and F. Stratman, eds.). Elsevier, New York, 1988; 415-426.

Lau, C.L., Slotkin, T.A., Molec. Pharmacol. (18), 1980; 247-252.

Lee S, Rivier C "Effect of postnatal exposure of female rats to an alcohol diet: influence of age and circulating sex steroids." Alcohol Clin Exp Res 1994 Aug;18(4):998-1003

Leighton, B.L., Tagliafero, A.R., J. Nutrition (117), 1987; 1287.

Lemmen, C., Barth, C.A., Wolfram, G., Zollner, N., Biochem. Biophys. ACTA. (755), 1983; 137-143.

Leonard, J.L., Kaplan, N.M., Visser, T.J., et al., Science (214), 571-573.

Lephart, E.D., Baxter, C.R., et al., J. Clin. Endocrinol. Netab. (64), 1987; 842-848.
Levesgue, W.A., Herzog, A.G., Seibel, N.M., J. Clin. Endocrinol. Metab (63), 1986; 243-245.

Levin, B.E., Triscari, J., Sullivan, A.C., Am. J. Physiol. (24), R170-R178.

Lewis, D.A., "Anti-inflammatory drugs from plant and marine sources." Agents Actions Suppl (27), 1989; 373.

Lipman, J.M., Turturro, A., Hart, R.W., Mech. Age Develop. (48), 1989; 135-143.
Li, K., Foo, T., Adams, J.B., Steroids (31), 1978; 113-127.

Li. K., Chandra, D.P., Foo, T., Steroids (28), 1976; 561-574.
Lipman, J.M., Turturro, A., Hart, R.W., Mech. Age Develop. (48), 1989; 135-143.

Lohman, T.G., "Skinfolds and body density and their relation to body fatness." Human Biol (53), 1991; 181-225.

Lohman, R., et al "DHEA protects muscle flap microcirculatory hemodynamics from ischemia/reperfusion injury; an experimental in vivo study." J Trauma. 1997;42:74-80.

London BM; Lookingbill DP "Frequency of pregnancy in acne patients taking oral antibiotics and oral contraceptives" [letter] Arch Dermatol 1994 Mar;130(3):392-3

Lookingbill, D.P., Egan, N., Santen, J., Demeres, L.M., J. Clin. Endocrinol. Metab. (67), 1988; 986-991.

Lopez, S.A., Wingo, C., Herbert, J.A., et al., Atherosclerosis. (24), 1976; 471-481.

Loria, R.M., Inge, T.H., Cook, et al., J. Med. Virol. (26), 1988; 301-314.

Lucas, J.A., Ahmed, S.A., Casey, N.L., MacDonald, P.C., J. Clin. Invest. (75), 1985; 2091-2093.

MacIndoe, J.H., Encodrinol. (123), 1988; 1281-1287.

Majewska, M.D., Demirgoren, S., Spivak, C.E., London, E.D., "The neurosteroid dehydroepiandrosterone sulfate is an allostericantagonist of the GABAA receptor." Brain Res 526(1), 1990 Aug 27; 143-146.

Malinow, M.R., Elliott, W.H., McLaughlin, P., Upson, B., "Effects of synthetic glycosides on steroid balance in Macacafascicularis." J. Lipid Res. 28(1), 1987 Jan; 1-9.

Mann, D.R., Castracane, V.D., McLaughlin, F., et al., Biol. Repro. 28, 279-284.

Marrero, M., Prough, R.A., Frenkel, R.A., Milewich, L., "Dehydroepiandrosterone feeding and protein phosphorylation, phosphatases, and lipogenic enzymes in mouse liver." Exp. Clin. Endocrinol 96(2), 1990 Nov; 149-156.

Martikainen, S., Heikkinen, J., Ruokonen, A., Kapuppila, A., J. Clin. Endocrinol. Metab. 66, 1988; 987-991.

Martin, S.N., Noberg, G.P., Life Sci. (29), 1981; 1683-1686.

Marynick, S.P., Chakmakjian, Z.H., McCaffree, D.L., Herndon, H., Jr. N. Engl. J. Med. (308), 1983; 981-986.

Matsumoto, A.M., "'Andropause'—are reduced androgen levels in aging men physiologically important?" West J Med, 1993 Nov; 159(5):618-620. Comment on: West J. Med, 1993 Nov; 159(5):579-585.

Mayer, D., Weber, E., Bannasch, P l, "Modulation of liver carcinogenesis by dehydroepiandrosterone. In the biological role of dehydroepiandrosterone." edited by M. Kalimi and W. Regelson, New York: deGruyter, 1990; 361-385.

Mayer, D., Weber, E., Moore, M.A., Carcinogenesis (9), 1988; 2039-2043.

Maynard, P.V., Bird, M., Basu, P.K., Brit. J. Cancer (14), 1978; 549-553.
Maynard, P.V., Pike, A.W., Weston, A., et al., Eur. J. Cancer (13), 1975; 971-975.

Melchior, C., Ritzmann, R.F., "Dehydroepiandrosterone is an anxiolytic in mice on the plus maze." Pharmacol Biochem Behav 47(3), 1994 Mar; 437-441.

Merril, C.R., Hanrington, M.G., Sunderland, T., "Reduced plasma dehydroepiandrosterone concentrations in HW infections and Alzheimer's disease. In the biological role of dehydroepiandrosterone." edited by Kalimi, M., and Regelson, W., New York: de Gruyter, 1990; 101-105.

Merriman, R.L., Tanzir, L.R., Stamm, N.B., et al., 13th Int. Cancer. Cong., Seattle, Washington, 1981.

Meyer, J.H., Gruol, D.L., "Dehydroepiandrosterone sulfate alters synaptic potentials in areas of CA1 of the hi pocampal slice." Maturitas, 17(3), 1993 Nov; 205-210.

Midgley, P.C., Azzopardi, D., Oates, N., Shat, J.C., Honour, J.W., "Virilisation of female preterm infants." Arch. Dis. Child 65(7 Spec No.), 1990 Jul; 701-703.

Milewich, L., Hendricks, T., Largelius, A., et al., Naturits (4), 1982; 113-118.

Mobbs, C.V., "Neurohormonal hysterisis as a mechanism for aging in humans and other species: comparative aspects development, maturation and senescence of neuroendocrine systems: a comparative approach." (M.P. Schreibman and C.G. Scanes, eds.), Academic Press, New York, 1989; 223-252.

Mochizuki, M., Tojo, S., "In: Dilation of the uterine cervix." (F. Naftolin and P.G. Stubblefield, eds. Raven Press, New York, 1980; 267-286.

Moffat, U., J. Amer. Dietetic. Assoc. (84), 1984;136.

Moise, J., Ilekis, J., Scommegna, A., Benveniste, R., Am. J. Obstet, Gynecol. (154), 1986; 1080-1085.

Monroe, S.E., Menon, K.M.J., "Changes in reproductive hormone secretion during the climacteric and postmenopausal periods." Clin Obstet Gynecol, 1977; 20:113-122.

Montanini, V., Simoni, N., Chiosse, G., et al., Horm. Res. (19), 1988; 1-6.

Morales, A.J., Nolan, J.J., Nelson, J.C., Yen, S.S., "Effects of replacement dose of dehydroepiandrosterone in men and women of advancing age." Eng. J. Clin. Endocrinol. Metab. 78(6), 1994 Jun; 1336-1340.

Motorola, J.F., and Yen, S.S.C., "The effects of oral dehydroepiandrosterone on endocrine-metabolic parameters in postmenopausal women." J Clin Endocrinol Metab, 1990; 71:696-704.

Moore, M.A., Weber, E., Thornton, M., et al Carcinogenesis (9), 1988; 1507-1059.

Mowrey, D.B., "Proven herbal blends." The Scientific Validation of Herbal Medicine, Keats Publishing, New Canaan, Conn., 1986; 19.

Murphy, S., Khaw, K.T., Cassidy, A., Compston, J.E., "Sex hormones and bone mineral density in elderly men." Bone Miner, 1993 Feb; 20(2):133-140.

Nagasaki, H., "Gender-related differences of mouse liver D-aspartate oxidase in the activity and response to administration of D-aspartate and peroxisome proliferators." Int. J. Biochem. 26(3), 1994 Mar; 415-423.

Nakamura, K.D., Duffy, P.H., CU, M.H., et al., Mech. Age Develop. (48), 1989; 199-205.

Natoli, C., Sica, G., Natoli, V., et al., J. Steroid Biochem. (15), 1981; 409-413.

Nawata H; Tanaka S; Tanaka S; et al "Aromatase in bone cell: association with osteoporosis in postmenopausal women." J Steroid Biochem Mol Biol 1995 Jun;53(1-6):165-74

Nestler, J.E., Beer, N.A., Jukubowicz, D.J., Beer, R.M., "Effects of a reduction in circulating insulin by metformin on serum dehydroepiandrosterone sulfate in nondiabetic men." J Clin Endocrinol Metab, 1994 Mar; 78(3):549-554.

Nestler, J.E., Clore, J.N., Strauss, J.F., III, Blackard, W.G., J Clin. Endocrinol. Metab. (64), 1987; 180-184.

Nestler, J.E., Clore, J.N., Blackard, W.G., "Metabolism and actions of dehydroepiandrosterone in humans." J Steroid Biochem Mol Biol, 1991; 40(6):599-605.

Nestler, J.E., Clore, J.N., Blackard, W.G., "Dehydroepiandrosterone: the missing link between hyperinsulinemia and atherosclerosis?: FASEB J, 1992 Sept; 6(12):3073-3075.

Nestler, J.E., Strauss, J.F., "Insulin as an effector of human ovarian and adrenal steroid metabolism." Endocrinol Metab Clin North Am, 1991 Dec; 20(4):807-823.

Nestler, J.E., Lisiskin, K.S., Barolascini, C.O., et al., J Clin. Endocrinol. Metab. (69), 1989; 1040-1046.

Nestler, J.E., McClanahan, M.A., "Diabetes and adrenal disease." Baillieres Clin Endocrinol Metab, 1992 Oct; 6(4):829-847.

Niort, G., Boccuzzi, G., et al., J. Steroid Biochem. (23), 1985; 657-661.

Nishi, Y., "Nonclassical 3 beta-hydroxysteroid dehydrosenase deficiency in young girls with hirsutism and premature pubarche." Endocrinol Jpn. 37(5), 1990 Oct; 763-767.

Nordin, B.E.C., et al., "The relation between calcium absorption, serum dehydroepiandrosterone, and vertebral mineral density in postmenopausal women." J. Clin. Endocrinol Metab., 1985; 60:651-657.

Nyce, J.W., et al., "Inhibition of 1,2-dimethylhydrazine induced colon tumeriogenesis in Balb/c mice by dehydroepiandrosterone." Carcinogenesis, 1984; 5:57-62.

Oberfield, S.E., Kairam, R., Bakshi, S., Bamji, M., Bhushan, et al "Steroid response to adrenocorticotropin stimulation in children with human immunodeficiency virus infection." J. Clin. Endocrinol Metab. 70(3), 1990 Mar; 578-581.

O'Brian, J., "Effect of diet on polyunsaturated fats on some platelet function tests." Lancet 2, 1976; 433.

O'Connell, Y., McKenna, T.J., Cunningham, S.K., "The effect of prolactin, human chorionic gonadotropin, insulin, and insulin-like growth factor 1 on adrenal steroidogenesis in isolated guinea-pig adrenal cells." J. Steroid Biochem. Mol. Biol. 48(2-3), 1994 Feb; 235-240.

Odumosu, A., Wilson, C.W., "Hypocholesterolemic effects of vitamin C, clofibrate and diosgenin in male guinea-pigs [proceedings]." Br. J. Pharmacol 67(3), 1979 Nov; 456P-457P.

Oertel, G.W., Teriber, L., Eur. J. Biochem. (7), 1969; 234-238.

O'Higgins, N.J., Carson, P., Mitchell, I., et al., Clin. Oncol. (2), 1976; 267-275.

Ohshima, K., Hayashi, N., Acta Obstet. Gynaecol. Jpn. (31), 1979; 1853-1861.

Oppenheimer, J.H., Mariash, C.N., Towle, et al., Life Sci. (28), 1981; 1693-1697.

Orentreich, N.J., Brind, L., Rizer, R.L., Vogelman, J.H., J. Clin. Endocrinol. Metab. (59), 1984; 551-555.

Orlandi, F., Carachi, P., Puligheddu, B., et al., "Estrone-3-sulfate in human breast cyst fluid. Relationship to cition-related cyst subpopulations." Ann. N Y Acad. Sci. 586, 1990; 79-82.

Oseko, F., Norikawa, K., Nakano, A., et al., Androloga (18), 1986; 523-528.

Oskai, L.B., "The role of exercise in weight control." In: Wilmore, J.H., ed. Exercise and Sport Science Reviews Vol (1), New York: Academic Press, 1975; 105-123.

Owasoyo, J.O., Bunike, G.N., Iramain, C.A., Endokrinologie. (77); 242-246.

Ozasa, H., Tominaga, Takeda, T., ACTA Obstet. Gynecol. Scand. (65), 1986; 543-545.

Ozasa, H., Tominaga, Nishimura, T., Takeda, J., Endocrinol. (109), 1981; 618-621.

Paczkowski, C., Wojciechowski, Z.A., "The in vitro synthesis of disogenin mono- and diglucoside by enzyme preparations from Solanum melongea leaves." Acta. Biochim. Pol. 40(1), 1993; 141-143.

Paolisso, G., "Metabolic features of patients with and without coronary heart disease but with a superimposable cluster of cardiovascular risk factors.: Coron Artery Dis, 1993 Dec; 4(12):1085-1091.

Parker, L.N., Levin, E.R., Lifrak, E.T., J. Endocrinol. Metab. (60), 1985; 947-951.

Parker, C.R., Jr., Leveno, K., et al., J. Clin. Endocrinol. Metab. (54), 1982; 1216-1220.

Parker, L., "Adrenal androgens in clinical medicine." Academic Press, New York, 1988.

Parker, C.R., Jr., Simpson, E.R., Bilheimer, D.W., et al., Science (206), 1980; 514-572.

Parker, Richard, et al *Journal of Trauma*, (1985) Vol 25, pg 508.

Paroli, G.C., Pantalioni, P., et al., Arch. Int. Pharm. Ther. (156), 1978; 147-150.

Pashiko, L.L., Schwartz, A.G., Agou-Gharbia, M., Carcinogenesis (46), 1981; 717-721.

Pashiko, L.L., Fairman, D.K., Schwartz, A.G., Gerontol. (41), 1986; 433-438.

Pashiko, L.L., Schwartz, A.G., Agou-Gharbia, M., Carcinogenesis (2), 1981; 717-721.

Paternostros, G., "Longevity and testosterone." [letter; comment] Nature, 1994 Mar 31; 368-(6470): 408 Comment on Nature, 1993 Nov 18; 366 (6452):215.

Pavlov, G.P., Harman, S.M., Chrousos, G.P., et al., J. Clin. Endocrinol. Metab. (62), 1986; 767-772.

Peh, K.L., Gunasegaram, R., Loganath, A., Horm. Metabol. Res. (19), 1987; 231-232.

Pepe, G.J., Waddell, B., Albreche, E.D., Endocrinol. (122), 1988; 646-650.

Perera, M.I.R., Shinozuka, H., Carcinogenesis (5), 1984; 1193-1198.

Piepaoli, W., Changxian, Y., J. Neuroimmunol., 1990.

Pitts, R.L., J. Am. Acad. Dermatol. (16), 1987; 571-573.

Prasad, V.V., Vegesna, S.R., Welch, M., Lieberman, S., "Precursors of the neurosteroids." Department of Obstetrics and Gynecology, Physiol. Behav. 55(2), 1994 Feb; 225-229.

Parough, R.A., Webb, S.J., Wu, H.Q., Lapenson, D.P., Waxman, D.J., "Induction of microsomal and peroxisomal enzymes by dehydroepiandrosterone and its reduced metabolite in rats." Cancer Res. 54(11), 1994 Jun 1; 2878-2886.

Puche, R.C., Romano, M.D., Tiss. Res (2), 1968; 133-144.

Purifoy, F.E., Koopinans, L.H., Tatuin, R.W., Human Biol. (52), 1980; 181-191.

Purohit, A., Howarth, N.M., Potter, B.V., Reed, M.J.m "Inhibition of steroid sulphatase activity by steroidal methylthiophosphonates: potential therapeutic agents in breast cancer." Metabolism 43(5), 1994 May; 599-603.

Ranke, N.B., Rosendahl, W., Gupta, D., Hormone Res. (16), 1982; 32-41.

Recordati, Informational Package, "Dehydroepiandrosterone industria chimica" I. Farmaceutica. s.p.a. Milano.

Reed MJ; Purohit A; Duncan LJ; et al "The role of cytokines and sulphatase inhibitors in regulating oestrogen synthesis in breast tumours." J Steroid Biochem Mol Biol 1995 Jun;53(1-6):413-20

Reff, M.E., Schneider, E.L., "Biological markers in aging." Bethesda, HIH.Pub., 1980; 82-2221.

Regelson, W., Loria, R., Kalimi, M.K., Ann. N. Acad. Sci. (521), 1988, 260-273.

Regelson, W., Pierpaoli, W., Cancer Investigation. (5), 1987; 379-385.

Regelson, W., "In: Intervention in the aging process." Part 2 (W. Regelson and N. Sinex, eds.) Alan R. Liss, New York, 1983; 3-52.

Regelson, W., Kalimi, M., "Dehydroepiandrosterone (DHEA) the multifunctional steroid. II. Effects on the CNS, cell proliferation, metabolic and vascular, clinical and other effects. Mechanism of action?" Medical College of Virginia, Virginia Commonwealth University, Richmond 23298.

Regelson, W., Loria, R., Kalimi, M., "Dehydroepiandrosterone (DHEA) the mother steroid. Immunologic action." Medical College of Virginia, Virginia Commonwealth University, Richmond 23298, Ann N Y Acad Sci (719), May 31, 1994; 553-563.

Regeleson, W., Leria, R., Kalimi, M., "Hormonal intervention: "buffer hormones" or state dependency. The role of dehydroepiandrosterone (DHEA), thyroid hormone, estrogen and hypophysectomy in aging." Ann N Y Acad Sci, 1988; 521:260-273.

Remer, T., Hintelmann, A., Manz, F., "Measurement of urinary androgen sulfates without previous hydrolysis: a tool to investigate adrenarche. Determination of total 17-ketosteroid sulfates." Research Institute of Child Nutrition, Dortmund, Germany. Report of National Institute of Health Expert Panel on Weight-loss. Meeting in Bethesda, MD, 31 March - 2 April 1992.

Risdon G; Cope J; Bennett M "Mechanisms of chemoprevention by dietary dehydroisoandrosterone. Inhibition of lymphopoiesis." Am J Pathol 1990 Apr;136(4):759-69

Rittmaster, R.S., Thompson, D.L., "Effects of leuprolide and dexamethasone on hair growth and hormone levels in hirsute women: the relative importance of the ovary and the adrenal in the pathogenesis of hirsutism." J. Clin. Endocrinol Metab. 70(4), 1990 Apr; 1096-1102.

Robel, P., Bourreau, E., Corpechot, C., et al., Steroid Biochem. (27), 1987; 649-655.

Rogers, W.N., Blaver, K.L., Beanton, W., Proc. Ain. Soc. Endocrinol. Abs (668), 1989; 189.

Rosen, T., Hansson, T., Granhed, H., Szucs, J., Bengtsson, B.A., "Reduced bone mineral content in adult patients with growth hormone deficiency." Acta Endocrinol(Copenh), 1993 Sept; 129(3):201-206.

Rosen, T., Eden, S., Larson, G., Wilhelmsen, L., Bengtsson, B.A., "Cardiovascular risk factors in adult patients with growth hormone deficiency." Acta Endocrinol(Copenh), 1993 Sep; 129(3):195-200.

Rowland, D.L., Greenleaf, W.J., Dorfman, L.J., Davidson, J.M., "Aging and sexual function in men." Arch Sex Behav, 1993 Dec 22; (6):545-557.

Rozenberg, S., et al. "Age, steroids and bone mineral content." Maturatis, 1990; 12:137-143.

Ruutianen, K., Erkkola, R., Gronroos, M.A., Kaihola, H.L., Fertl. and Sterility (50), 1988; 255-259.

Sadowsky, M., Antonovsky, H., Sobel, R., Maoz, B., "Sexual Activity and sex hormone levels in aging men." Int Psychogeriatrics, 1993 Fall; 5(2):181-186.

Sakyo, K., Ito, A., Mori, Y., J. Pharmacobiodyn. (9), 1986; 276-286.

Sakyo, K., Ito, A., Mori, Y., Biol. Repro. (36), 1987; 277-281.

Sakyo, K., Ito, A., Ogawa, C., Mori, Y., Biophys, Acta. (883), 1986; 517-522.

Sambrotk, P.N., et al., "Sex hormones status and osteoporosis in postmenopausal women with rheumatoid arthritis." Arthritis Rheum, 1988; 31:973-978.

Sasagawa, I., Satomi, S., "Effects of high-dose medroxyprogesterone acetate on plasma hormone levels and pain relief in patients with advanced prostatic cancer." Br. J. Urol. 65(3), 1990 Mar; 278-281.

Schiebinger, R., Chrousous, G.P., Cutler, G.B., Jr., Lorianux, D.C., J. Clin. Endocrinol. Metab. (62), 1986; 202-209.

Schmidt, J.B., Lindmaier, A., Spona, J., "Endocrine parameters in ance vulgaris." Department of Dermatology II, University of Vienna, Austria, Endocrinol Exp. 24(4), 1990 Dec; 457-464.

Schubert W, Cullberg G, Edgar B, Hedner T "Inhibition of 17 beta-estradiol metabolism by grapefruit juice in ovariectomized women." Maturitas 1994 Dec;20(2-3):155-63.

Schulz S; Nyce JW "Inhibition of protein isoprenylation and p21ras membrane association by dehydroepiandrosterone in human colonic adenocarcinoma cells in vitro." Cancer Res 1991 Dec 15;51(24):6563-7

Schwartz, A.G., Pashko, L.L., "Cancer chemoprevention with the adrenocortical steroid dehydroepiandrosterone & structural analogs." J Cell Biochem Suppl (17G), 1993; 73-79.

Schwartz, A.G., Fairman, D.K., et al., "The biological significance of dehydroepiandrosterone." Carcinogenesis (10), 1988; 1809.

Schwartz, A.G., "Inhibitions of spontaneous breast cancer formation in female C3H(Avy'a) mice aby long-term treatment with dehydroepiandrosterone." Cancer Res, 1979; 39:1129-1132.

Schwartz, A.G., Whitcomb, J., et al., Adv. Cancer Res. (51), 1988; 391-424.

Seiger, A., and A.C. Granholm. Cell Tissue Res., 1981; 1-15.

Selye, Hans, M.D., "The stress of life." McGraw Hill, New York, NY, 1984.

Semple, C.G., Gray, C.E., Bearstall, Acta Endocrinol. (Copenhag). (116), 1987; 155-160.

Sengupta SN, Ray R, et al "Pituitary gonadal functioning in male alcoholics in an Indian psychiatric hospital." Alcohol Alcohol 1991;26(1):47-51.

Shenfield GM Oral contraceptives. "Are drug interactions of clinical significance? " Drug Saf 1993 Jul;9(1):21-37

Shapiro, M.S., Zelefsky, S., Chayen, R., Werber, M.M., J. Clin. Chem. Clin. Biochem. (27), 1989; 27-31.

Shikata, J., Sanada, H., Yamamuro, T. et al, Connect. Tissue Res. (7), 1979; 21-27.

Shimomura, Y., Bray, G.A., Kee, N., Horm. Metabol. Res. (19), 295-299.

Short, S.H., "Dietary surveys and nutrition knowledge." In: Hickson, J.F., Wolinsky, I., eds. Nutrition in Exercise and Sport. Boca Raton, FL: CRC Press, 1989; 309-343.

Sica, G., Natoli, C., Narchetti, P., et al., J. Steroid Biochem (15), 1981; 415-419.

Siegel, S.F., Finegold, D.N., Lanes, R., Lee, P.A., "ACTH stimulates tests and plasma dehydroepiandrosterone sulfate levels in women with hirsutism." N. Engl. J. Med. 323(13), 1990 Sept 27; 909-911, and N. Eng. I. Med 324(8), 1991 Feb 21; 5645 and Metabolism 39(9), 1990 Sept; 967-970.

Siegler, J.M., N.N. Kazalrinoff. Nutr. & Cancer. (4), 1983; 176-180.

Simard, J., Vincent, A., Duchesne, R., Labrie, F., Mol. Cell Endocr. (55), 1988; 233-242.

Simunova, 3., Gregorova, I., Soiska, J., "Metabloicke komplekace otylosti-poloss oje-jich ovbmmi denydroeptandrosteron sulfatem." Steroik Uk., 1973; (75) 27-30.

Smith, C.P., Dunger, D.B., Williams A.J.K., et al., J. Clin. Endocrinol. Metab. (68), 1989; 932-938.

Spivak, C.E./, "Desensitization and noncompetitive blockage of GABAA receptors inventral midbrain neurons by a neurosteroid dehydropiandrosterone sulfate." Addiction Research Center, National Institute on Drug Abuse, Baltimore, Maryland. Sonka, J., ACTA Univ. Carol (71), 1971; 1-137, 146-171.

Sonka, J., et al., "Defecit des dehydroepiandrosterone nenee syndrome?" Endocrinology, 47, 1965; 152-161.
Sonka, J., Stravkova, M., Aggressologie (5), 1970; 421-426.

Sonka, J., et al., "Serum lipids and dehydroepiandrosterone excretion in normal sub-jects." Journal of Lipid Research, 9, 1968; 769-772.

Steen, S.N., McKinney, S., Physician & Sports Med (14), 1986; 100.

Strauss, E.B., Psychotherapie U. Med Psychologie. (5), 1955; 2-10.

Sulcova, J., Starka, L., Jirasek, J.E., Endocrinol. Exp. (16), 1982; 9-17.

Sulman, F.G., American Lecture Series, Thomas, Springfield, Ill., 1980.

Sun, X. R., Risbrider, G.P., "Site of macropage inhibition of luteinizing hormone-stimulated testosterone production by purified leydig cells." Biol Reprod 50(2), 1994 Feb; 363-367.

Sunderland, T., Nerril, C.R., Harrington, M.G., "DHEA and Alzheimer's disease." Lancet (2), 1989; 570.

Svec, F., Lopez, S., Lancet II, 1989; 1335-1336.

Taelman, P., et al., "Persistence of increased bone resorption and possible role of dehydroepiandrosterone as a bone metabolism determinant in osteoporotic women in late postmenopause." Maturitas, 1989; 11:65-73.

Tandon, A.K., Clark, G.M., et al., N. Engl J. Med. (322), 1990; 297-302.

Tauber, U., Weiss, C., Matthes, H., "Does salicylic acid increase and percutaneous absorption of diflucortolone-21-valerate?" Skin Pharmacol 6(4), 1993; 276-281.

Tegelman, R., Carlstrom, K., Pousette, A., Int. J. Androl. (11), 1988; 361-368.

Thewles, A., Parslow, R.A., Coleman, R., "Effect of diosgenin on biliary cholesterol transport in the rat." Bioiichem J. 291 (Pt3), 1993 May 1; 793-798.

Thomas, B.S., Kirby, P., Ses, E.E., Wang, D.Y., Europ. J. Cancer (12), 1976; 405-409.

Tipton, C.M., Physicians & Sports Med. (15), 1987; 160.

Tipton, C.M., Olinger, R.A., Iowa Medicine (74), 1984; 381.

Tomic, R., Ljungberg, B., Damber, J.E., Scand. J. Urol. Nephrol. (72), 1988; 15-18.

Torti, F.M., Dieckmann, B., Beutier, B., Science (221), 1985; 867-869.

Toth, I., Faredin, I., Acta Med. Hung. (40), 1983; 139-145.

Tourney, G., Hatfield, L.M., Arch. Gen Psychiat. (27), 1972; 753-755.

Tourney, G., Hatfield, L.M., Biol. Psych. (6), 1973; 23-26.

Uchida, K., Takase, H., Nomura, Y., Takeda, K., et al, "Changes in bilary and fecal bile acids in mice after treatments with diosgenin and beta-sitosterol." J. Lipid Res. 25(3), 1984 Mar; 236-245.

US News and World Report (3), February 1992; 55-60.

Utsuonmiya, T., Sumioki, H., Taniguchi, I., "Hormonal and clinical effects of multi-follicular puncture and resection on the ovaries of polycystic ovary syndrome." J Rheumatol (3), 1994 Mar 21; 430-434.

Valimaki MJ, Laitinen K, Tiitinen A, et al "Gonadal function and morphology in non-cirrhotic female alcoholics: a controlled study with hormone measurements and ultrasonography." Acta Obstet Gynecol Scand 1995 Jul;74(6):462-6.

Valimaki M, Pelkonen R, et al "Pituitary-gonadal hormones and adrenal androgens in non-cirrhotic female alcoholics after cessation of alcohol intake." Eur J Clin Invest 1990 Apr;20(2):177-81.

Van Landeghem, A.A.J., Poortinan, J., Nabuurs, M., Thijssen, J.H.H., Cancer Res. (45), 1985; 2907-2912.

Van Noorden, C.J., Vogels, I.C.M., Houtkooper, J.M., et al., Eur. J. Cell Biol. (33), 1984; 157-162.

Vermeulen, A., Ando, S., Clin Endocrinol. (8), 1978; 295-303.

Vilette, J.M., et al., "Circadian variations in plasma levels of hypophyseal, adrenocortical and testicular hormones in men infected with human immunodeficiency virus." Comment in: J. Clin. Endocrinol Metab. 70(3), 1990 Mar; 563-565, and J. Clin Endocrinol Metab 70(3), 1990 Mar; 572-577.

Wade, C.E., Lindberg, J.S., Cockerell, J.L., et al., J. Clin. Endocrinol. Metab. (67), 1988; 223-227.

Walsh, S.W., Obstet. Gynecol. (71), 1988; 222-226.

Watson, A.Y., Radie, K., McCarthy, N., et al., Endocrinol. (110, 1392-1401.

Wang, D.Y., Bulbrook, R.D., Herian, M., et al., Eur. J. Cancer (10), 1974; 477-482.

Ward, R.C., Costoff, A., Nahesh, V.B., Biol. Reprod. (18), 1978; 614-623.

Warren, N.P., Brooks-Gunn, J., J. Clin Endocrinol. Metab. (68), 1989; 77-83.

Watters, J.M., Besey, P.Q., Dinarello, C.A., et al., Surgery (98), 1985; 289-306.

Weber, E., Moore, M.A., et al, Carcinogenesis (9), 1988; 1049-1054, 1191-1195.

Whitcomb. J. M. et al DHEA inhibit 12-O tetrdecanoylphorbol-13-acetate stimulation of superoxide radical production by phuman polymorphocuclear leukocytyes." Carcinogenosis 1985, 6: 333-335

Wiebe, R.H.S., Handwerber, J Repro. Med. (28), 1983; 206-208.

Wild, R.A., Buchanen, J.R., et al., Proc. Soc. Exp. Biol. Med. (186), 1987; 355-360.

Wilmore, J.H., "Body composition in sport and exercise: directions for future research." Med. Sci. Sports Exer. (15), 1983; 21-31.

Wilpart, M., Speder, A., Ninane, P., Roberfroic, M., Teratogenesis Carcinogenesis, Mutagenesis. (6), 1986; 265-273.

Wimalasena J, Beams F Caudle MR " Ethanol modulates the hormone secretory responses induced by epidermal growth factor in choriocarcinoma cells. " Alcohol Clin Exp Res 1994 Dec;18(6):1448-55

Wise T; Klindt J; Buonomo FC "Obesity and dehydroepiandrosterone/ dehydroepiandrosterone sulfate relationships in lean, obese, and meat-type cross-bred boars: responses to porcine growth hormone." Endocrinology 1995 Aug;136(8):3310-7

Yamaji, T., Ishibashi, N., Takau, F., et al., Acta Endocriniol (Copenh)(120), 1989; 655-660.

Yamamoto, A., Serizawa, S., Ito, M., Sato, Department of Dermatology, Niigata University School of Medicine, Japan, J. Dermatol Sci. 1(4), 1990 Jul; 269-276.

Yang JY; Schwartz A; Henderson EE "Inhibition of 3'azido-3'deoxythymidine-resistant HIV-1 infection by dehydroepiandrosterone in vitro." Biochem Biophys Res Commun 1994 Jun 30;201(3):1424-32

Yang JY; Schwartz A; Henderson EE "Inhibition of HIV-1 latency reactivation by dehydroepiandrosterone (DHEA) and an analog of DHEA." AIDS Res Hum Retroviruses 1993 Aug;9(8):747-54

Yen SS, Murphy AA, Kettel LM,. Morales AJ, Roberts VJ "Regression of uterine leiomyomata in response to the antiprogesterone RU 486." J Clin Endocrinol Metab 1993 Feb;76(2):513-7

Yen SS, Morales AJ, Nolan Nelson, JC.,"Effects of replacement dose of dehydroepiandrosterone in men and women of advancing age." J Clin Endocrinol Metab 1994 Jun;78(6):1360-7

Yen, T.T., et al., "Prevention of obesity in Avy'a mice by dehydroepian. drosterone." Lipid, 1977; 12:409-413.

Yuen, B.H., Mincey, E.K., Am. J. Obstet. Gynecol. (156), 1978; 396-400.

Zambraski, E., et al., Med. Scil Sports (8), 1976; 105.

Zuidema, L.J., Knan-Dawood, F., Dawood, N.Y., Work, B.A., Jr., Am. J. Obstet. Gynecol. (155), 1986; 1252-1254.

Zumoff, B., Walsh, T., et al., J. Clin. Endocrinol. Metab. (56), 1983; 672-676.

Zumoff, B., Levin, J., Rosenfled, S., et al., "Abnormal 24-hr mean plasma concentrations of dehydroepiandrosterone and dehydroepiandrosterone sulfate in women with in- operable breast cancer." Cancer Res. (41), 1981; 3360-3363.

# INDEX

# YOU NEED TO KNOW...
## THE HEALTH MESSAGE

*I Corinthians 3:16-17*
Do you not know that you are God's temple and that God's Spirit dwells in you? If any one destroys God's temple, God will destroy him, For God's temple is holy and that temple you are.

---

## Health Learning Handbooks

**Castor Oil: Its Healing Properties**
by Beth Ley  36 pages, $3.95

**Dr. John Willard on Catalyst Altered Water**
By Beth Ley  60 pages, $3.95

**Colostrum: Nature's Gift to the Immune System**
By Beth Ley  80 pages, $4.95

**How to Fight Osteoporosis and Win! The Miracle of Microcrystalline Hydroxyapatite**
By Beth Ley  80 pages, $6.95

**The Potato Antioxidant: Alpha Lipoic Acid**
By Beth Ley  112 pages, $6.95

## Additional Titles

**Natural Healing Handbook**
by Beth Ley with foreword by Dr. Arnold J. Susser, R.P., Ph.D.  320 pages, $14.95

**How Did We Get So Fat?**
By Dr. Arnold J. Susser and Beth Ley, 96 pages, $7.95

**A Diet For The Mind**  By Fred Chapur, 112 pages, $8.95

**DHEA: Unlocking the Secrets of the Fountain of Youth- 2nd Edition**  By Beth Ley and Dr. Richard Ash 256 pages, $14.95

---

## TO ORDER:

Send check or money order to
BL Publications, 21 Donatello, Aliso Viejo, CA 92656
Please include $2.00 for shipping.

To order by credit card call toll free: **1-888-367-3432**